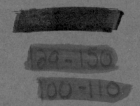

Joanna Kitt

Survey of
Communication Disorders

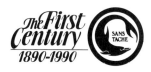

The First Century 1890-1990 · SANS TACHE

Survey of
Communication
Disorders

John M. Palmer, Ph.D.

Phillip A. Yantis, Ph.D.

Department of Speech and Hearing Sciences
University of Washington
Seattle, Washington

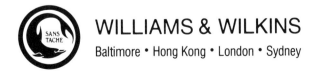

WILLIAMS & WILKINS
Baltimore • Hong Kong • London • Sydney

Editor: John P. Butler
Associate Editor: Linda Napora
Project Editor: Linda Hansford
Designer: Bob Och
Illustration Planner: Wayne Hubbel
Production Coordinator: Adèle Boyd-Lanham

Copyright (c) 1990
Williams & Wilkins
428 East Preston Street
Baltimore, Maryland 21202, USA

Printed in the United States of America

Library of Congress Cataloging-in-Publication Data
Palmer, John M. (John Milton), 1922–
    Survey of communication disorders / John M. Palmer, Phillip A. Yantis.
      p. cm.
    ISBN 0-683-06743-5
    1. Communicative disorders.   I. Yantis, Phillip A. II. Title.
    [DNLM: 1. Communicative Disorders. WL 340 P174s]
RC423.P22 1990
DNLM/DLC
for Library of Congress
                                              89-22411
                                                  CIP

90 91 92 93 94
1   2   3   4   5   6   7   8   9   10

Preface

This is an introductory book—a survey of the profession. Our subject is communication disorders, which are conditions that interfere with the usual efficiency with which people talk to people. Oral communication is accomplished through speech, hearing, and language. Both the normal and the disordered conditions of these important human functions are explored in this text.

Over our nearly 70 years of combined teaching experience, we have been impressed by the ever-increasing body of scientific knowledge associated with communication disorders. Our goal here has been to explore as much of that body of knowledge as is necessary to acquaint readers with the fundamentals of the topic. Although we have refrained from discussing the more intricate details of this complex subject, we have introduced the major facts underlying both normal and disordered oral communication and have suggested sources for further study. For example, we have referred to the development of language in children, to the structure and function of the human speech apparatus and the amazing inner ear, and to voice, language, and auditory disorders, among other topics.

We have recognized that many beginning students may be unprepared to examine such detailed topics as, for example, the development of object permanence in language acquisition, or the neural innervation of the vocal folds, or differential hair cell functions in the cochlea. Instead of detailed topics, we have tried to present essential features. Of course, superficial treatment of knowledge rarely satisfies the scientist—but that was not our goal. We blue-penciled and reduced content (advised in part by five classes of students who freely provided detailed feedback on earlier versions of the text) to preserve our target of presenting a broad scientific base. We have long been aware that some students prefer this degree of coverage as they prepare for careers in other professions, such as teaching or nursing. We have tried to serve them.

The "majors" in the field need not be concerned about superficiality in a text of this type. For those who plan to continue as advanced students (or who might become interested enough to explore that option) and will study beyond the scope of a survey course, our topic outline may be taken as representative; succeeding courses will amplify what is introduced herein. We are not concerned that this text be a complete compendium of knowledge in the field. By foreshortening detailed descriptions of scientific fact, we gained the freedom to discuss other aspects, particularly the human and professional implications of communication disorders. We point to education limitations, to self-esteem decrements, and to vocational problems. Brief clinical illustrations of fictional persons are composite examples drawn from our years of clinical experience. We introduce the field of speech-language pathology and audiology as a vocational choice.

Chapter 1 further explores the purposes of this text and discusses basic terminology, which is amplified in the Glossary. Following this background, we plunge into the individual topics associated with disorders of human communication.

We hope our goals are met. It is our desire that readers' personal interest in the helping professions of speech-language pathology and audiology will be stimulated. We hope further that we have explained the most human of all human behaviors—oral communication—and that we have provided a better understanding of the varied implications associated with disorders of this critical function.

John M. Palmer
Phillip A. Yantis

Acknowledgments

We express our deep appreciation and gratitude to those who have contributed to this writing.

To the many students who earlier struggled with one of the authors (JMP) as he adapted one of more than a dozen "survey" texts for use in an introductory course. Those students stimulated the effort to produce this book.

To our colleagues on the faculty of the Department of Speech and Hearing Sciences at the University of Washington. Knowing our many weaknesses, they enlightened us in many relevant matters. Where the material is accurate, correct, and clear, we thank them. Where we retained our errors and confusion, we accept responsibility. Faculty members who have been particularly helpful are Lesley Olswang, Alan Reich, Robert Carpenter, Truman Coggins, Charles Flowers, Gary Thompson, Ed Burns, Richard Folsom, and especially William Tiffany.

To the students who enthusiastically and generously contributed to this writing, especially Nathan Batuschek, Christine Buzard, Patricia Bjarnason, Verna Kilic, Mark Drake, Jackie Angvall, and Megan Blaumer.

We also thank Phyllis Wood, of Phyllis Wood Associates in Seattle, for the original artwork. Most of all, we acknowledge the patience, contribution, and skills of Arlene Chaussee in her direction of word processing. Many thanks.

Contents

1

About This Book and Its Topic

INTRODUCTION

This book was written for those with little or no knowledge about disordered human communication. It can accompany a lecture course, in which much of its content can be supplemented with suitable examples and illustrations in class meetings, or it can stand alone as an initial source of information for the inquiring reader who needs basic information. We have attempted to provide a motivational experience, encouraging further exploration into the field of communicative impairments. As a survey text, this book addresses the major, more common, most significant of the disorders experienced by human speakers and listeners. First, it is necessary to lay the foundations of the normal functioning or form that may be disordered; one must understand "normal" to understand "abnormal."

The various forms of disordered communication are many. Some have a rather uncomplicated nature that can be treated adequately in relatively limited ways. Others are rather complex, requiring exploration on a multidimensional scale. As noted above, all require some understanding of the normal aspects of communication from which the disorders vary. We also have tried to provide some insight into the implications of these disorders for the individual human life.

The content represents common knowledge and professional activity within speech-language pathology and audiology at the time of this writing. The emphases and involvement of those who provide services to the communicatively impaired will certainly change over the years. Suggested Readings included in each chapter provide sources for appropriate amplification. Some of these references represent other survey texts, some more specialized references, and still others are selected articles in professional journals showing the detail and depth often available in such sources. Any sources specifically referred to in the text are included in the Suggested Readings. The content was also designed to respond to the curiosity of those who may choose to begin the study of communication disorders. But whether this text serves as a launching pad or simply to broaden the reader's perspective of the human condition, we hope that it amplifies the critical importance of effective oral communication in human life.

To add some zest and challenge to the writing, we have included at the end of each chapter a series of Study Questions. These may not appear to be deep or scholarly, but they are intended to encourage the reader to consider practical, social, or personal aspects of the subject matter. They could become interesting examination questions.

HUMAN COMMUNICATION

Although often taken for granted, the ability of people to talk with each other is a uniquely human behavior. Other forms of animal and even botanical life provide stimuli of various forms to others of their kind: birds signal the presence of food or of the predator hawk; moose trumpet mating calls or make territorial announcements; certain trees even signal to others the presence of noxious and potentially dangerous chemicals. But the propositional communicative behavior referred to in this text is considered unique to the human being. It is a basic and necessary ingredient of expected social interaction. As such, it is one of the most important forms of human behavior. It differs significantly from the communicative behaviors of other creatures.

Humans communicate with others about the present, as do other living creatures. But the complexity of language usage and intellectual capacity allow communicative attention to matters of the past and future as well. Human communication is not bound by time. It is not limited to the "here and now."

Humans communicate by means of abstract concepts. They are not restricted to concrete matters such as food, danger, and mating behaviors. The state of the world, the nature of art, religion, personal attitudes and opinions—even the nature of communication disorders—all are appropriate subject matter for people talking with people. Human communication is propositional.

Humans communicate with others to exert dominance in many ways. Without resorting to physical force, humans can cause a change in the physical or mental condition of another through the simple act of oral communication. Humans can start a war, or stop it, through the avenue of spoken language. Cooperation can be fostered, or disrupted. Feelings of warmth and happiness can be stimulated in others, as can fear and insecurity. Human communication is relational.

The importance of oral communication to the definition of what is "human," then, is of utmost importance. Human communicative behavior is so integral to the natural state of our lives that it is hardly noticed or unusually appreciated as a skill—unless it is lost, or does not develop adequately. Human communication has several modalities. We can write and we can read. We can gesture or use sign language, and we can translate the meaning. Most commonly, however, we talk, we listen, and we "think" using language and speech. This book considers the basic aspects associated with common or normal oral communication and presents descriptions of variation from the normal in the major communication disorders categories.

About Terminology

The word "disorder" is commonly used to refer to a disturbance in the normal function or operation of something. As such, it requires an understanding of normality, of "order." Although "disorder" is popular as a term describing problems of human physiology, other terms are often used in similar contexts. The word "impairment" is an example. We must be circumspect, though, about our use of some common terms.

"Defect," "anomaly," "abnormality," and "deformity" are terms often used to describe irregularities, imperfections, and deviations from the norm, frequently in relation to anatomy or physiology. Similarly, the words "difference" and "variation" appear in discussions of observed changes in form, condition, or appearance as compared with some "normal" standard. "Handicap" is another common term. However, it suggests a condition that *results* from a disorder or impairment. It does not necessarily refer to the problem itself. A handicapping condition results in a negative influence on a person's life-style, creating unusual difficulty in achieving normal expectations in daily living. It is possible, of course, to have a disorder without a handicap. An example is a person with fewer (or perhaps more) than the usual complement of toes or fingers, who may still be entirely capable of performing efficiently the daily tasks expected of most individuals.

Where is the borderline between normal function or behavior and that which is labeled as a significant difference? People are not at all alike, either in physiology or in behavior. At what point do we identify variance as sufficiently large to label it as a "disorder"? What are the criteria used to identify differences in communicative skill as "abnormalities" or "disorders"? When is the oral communication skill of a person sufficiently different to be labeled disordered?

About Communication Disorders

We will define a "communication disorder" as *an observed disturbance in the normal speech, language, or hearing process.* We must add important qualifiers as presented by Dr. Charles Van Riper. One or more of three criteria must be in operation to identify a person's communication skills as disordered. These criteria are not entirely measurable or quantitative. They may be judgmental and subjective. They are not ordered; that is, one criterion is not more or less important to the definition than another. A person with disordered communication abilities may be so judged by a single criterion or by all three in combination and to varying degrees.

The three criteria are (1) objective signs, (2) social signs, and (3) personal signs. The use of the term "sign," borrowed from the medical lexicon, is an attempt to be objective, if not quantitative. In medical practice, the diagnostic physician examines two sets of conditions. One set is the symptom. This is the complaint expressed by the patient. It is sometimes reported in words such as hurt, pain, irritation, hot, cold, dizzy, and the like. There are some diagnostic strategies that attempt to objectify such terms, like rating scales. But it is extremely difficult to be sure that a condition causing a certain degree of pain to one person would have the same effect in another; one person's "dizziness" is not necessarily an experience similar to that of others who use the same term. The word "symptom," then, must be used cautiously.

A sign, however, is a term indicating that another person has observed a condition of interest, and may even be able to measure it. Medical practitioners measure a person's "fever" with a thermometer. Similarly, audiologists scale "hearing loss" with a device called an audiometer. Visual skills can be quantified, as can several bodily forms and functions. These measurements can then be used in making comparisons with what is known about average, normal characteristics. Signs and symptoms both are extremely important to the clinician, but it is necessary to recognize which of the two is being examined and to value each accordingly.

OBJECTIVE SIGNS

These communicative characteristics may be observed by another person. They are usually measurable. Some quantifiable difference exists that places specific behavior outside the range of normal. Objective signs may be seen in the sound-receiving system (audition), in the coding system (language), or in the sound-generating system (speech). Assume for an example that a person's voice is observed to be extremely high in frequency, or "high-pitched." If this person happens to be a large, muscular football player on a professional team, such communicative behavior would typically be considered "nonstandard" for adult males of similar physique. The vocal output could be measured acoustically by a variety of clinical instruments. The objective sign, then, would be the acoustic output of the subject's speech. Another objective sign is the result of measuring, audiometrically, an individual's hearing sensitivity.

SOCIAL SIGNS

What is the effect of a communication difference on other persons in the social environment? It is possible that others fail to understand the speaker's meaning and respond inappropriately, and mutual embarrassment may easily result. Another reaction is to ignore or avoid the speaker, or to withdraw from the speaker's presence as soon as possible. The effect of these behaviors in the mind of the speaker could lead to various interpretations: discrimination or punishment. The outcome is social failure.

PERSONAL SIGNS

This criterion refers to the speaker's own reaction to a self-perceived "disorder." Does the person withdraw from communicative activities? Do changes result in the home and work environment, including association with those once called friends? An individual with a developing hearing loss could find it difficult to be employed in work that involves considerable telephone usage, or answering questions of customers, or sales activity. Such a person might find it easier to move to other forms of employment where auditory skills carry less of a premium.

In all three criteria discussed above, it is obvious that communication disorders vary in their importance. Significant differences may be more noticeable to the speaker than to the listener, or vice versa. A simple example: for an agricultural fieldworker, a noticeable lisp might well create no vocational problem whatever. But a lisp, no matter how slight, could be extremely important and detrimental to an individual in radio broadcasting, or in sales, or in teaching. In a college drama class, a young man with such a lisp, ordinarily minor in degree, could be severely threatened by a drama coach judging such a difference as professionally detrimental.

PREVALENCE OF COMMUNICATION DISORDERS

It is inevitable when viewing a profession, and the people it serves, to ask, "How many?" Are only few people needing such services, with consequent restrictions in personnel to serve such a population? Alternatively, are the needs so great that the supply of professionals is insufficient? Such questions have practical implications for those having vocational interests in a profession.

Statistics relating to the communicatively impaired come from various sources. The federal government, state, and local health, welfare, and education agencies, private practitioners, and others carry out periodic surveys of specific populations. For example, all children in the first, third, and fifth grades in a certain school district might be included in annual speech-language-hearing screening programs, but such screening might not be done in private institutions. Figures utilized by the federal government are usually based on direct contact with a limited data base. Statistical extrapolation then occurs to estimate incidence in the general population. Therefore, at any point in time the statistics in this field are only estimates. Even so, they provide useful guidelines about the extent of communication disorders in our society.

The American Speech-Language-Hearing Association's brochures and journals lead us to believe that about 10% of the population in the United States has some form of communication impairment. At the time of this writing, we are referring to 23–24 million individuals of all ages. The same sources provide some prevalence figures for a few of the most common communication disorders. Problems associated with the production of speech sounds (consonants and vowels), including the voice, constitute the largest group (about 5%, or 11–12 million persons). Language disorders (those associated with grammar, syntax, etc., but not foreign language or dialect influences) constitute about 1%, or somewhat over 2 million people. Included in this number are children who have not yet learned language skills, as well as those who have modified skills after brain injury or other problems. Less than 1% of persons in the United States are said to be stutterers. Hearing disorders are problems that do not lend themselves to accurate statistical reporting. However, according to the American Speech-Language-Hearing Association, public health and educational screening programs show that about 4% of the population has communication disorders due to hearing impairment. Clearly, many more than this may have mild hearing losses, or impairments in only one ear. Some estimate about 2 million persons in the special category: deafness.

It appears, then, that there may be 23–24 million persons in the United States who are known to have some form of communication disorder. If more accurate demographic techniques could be applied, there is reason to believe that the figure would be considerably greater than this. This is a large portion of our population, and an important professional group had developed to serve these individuals.

TYPES OF DISORDERS

The prevalence of various disorders is difficult to measure, in part because of unclear definitions. To dispel some degree of ambiguity as we embark on our topic, we provide the following as our working definitions.

Speech disorders are variations from commonly used speech events in the acoustic character of the utterances one makes. This refers to the nature of the sounds we make as we talk, rather than to their meaning. Let us consider some examples.

We will see later that the voice is produced at the vocal folds and is resonated in the pharynx, nose, and mouth above. It is articulated (formed into speech sounds, or phonemes) by the movement of mouth structures, and subsequently flows smoothly as syllables and words as the speaker expresses ideas. Disorders may occur in any of these aspects.

Problems localized at the vocal folds may disturb voice production (phonation). These may be due to habit, physical changes in structure, or other problems associated with vocal fold function. Such a voice disorder is known as dysphonia. Vocal sounds are resonated in the chambers above the vocal folds. Most of the time this product is adequate, or even beautiful as in the case of an operatic soprano. At times, however, the resonance is affected by a cold or some other anatomic change. Many authorities classify resonance disorders as an extension of voice disorders—simply another subclass of the same voice production activity.

The resonated vocal sound is delivered into the oral cavity and is molded into the several speech sounds of our language; this is *articulation.* Movements of the anatomic parts maneuver the exhaled air as well as the resonated vocal sound to produce unique speech sounds (vowels and consonants). Disorders affecting the function of the articulators may cause unusual formation (or omission) of some speech sounds. This problem is one of the more common disorders of communication.

One of the most well-known categories of expressive communication disorder is stuttering. It is a speech disorder characterized by an interruption in the flowing speech. The interruption can be a pause, a repetition of a sound or word, or a prolongation of a sound. Not only does it interfere with communication, stuttering may cause important personality differences in the stutterer.

Language disorders are those involving the linguistic aspects of oral communication. The meaning, communicative intent, and linguistic code of the utterance cannot be conveyed successfully. Language disorders may be described in terms of the linguistic dimensions in which they fall. Thus, they may occur as semantic or meaningful disorders. They may be defined as pragmatic or use problems. We might describe them as syntactic or structural problems, that is, in the grammatical and phonologic dimensions of language. Each of these will be further explained in chapter 2. But language disorders may also be described according to the process used in the linguistic activity. Thus, we may find expressive problems found largely in the talking aspect, and receptive language problems, difficulties in understanding. We find recall or central brain-processing difficulties that are linguistic in nature.

These language disorders may be found in the developing years of childhood, as the child succeeds or fails in learning to speak the language spoken in the cultural environment. Language disorders also occur in the adult who has lost linguistic skills, perhaps as the result of some brain injury. In general, we are not referring to such problems in a person who is learning a specific language (e.g., an American learning German or Chinese) for the first time.

Hearing disorders stem from problems within the auditory system. Although this usually is associated with the ear, it may also be centered in the auditory receptor areas of the brain where the perception of word meanings and associations occur. The child with an ear infection may well suffer from a hearing disorder (on a very temporary basis, one hopes). An elderly person, on the other hand, may develop a hearing impairment slowly with advancing age as changes occur in the sensory cells of the inner ear. Irreversible impairment can occur following unusual levels of noise exposure. Growths, injuries, and infections may affect the neurologic aspects of the auditory system. Such factors can easily lead to serious difficulties in the ability to perceive and understand the speech of others.

SUMMARY

This textbook is intended to accompany a lecture/demonstration course survey-ing the various disorders of human communication or to serve readers curious about this subject. As a survey textbook, it does not delve deeply into any one aspect of the subject matter; it provides an introduction to the variety of disorders encompassed in the field. The reader should understand that disorders are a functional variation in what is known about normal communication processes. Both normal and disordered commu-nication are constantly under study and investigation. Advanced coursework and study will lead the student into a deeper study of nearly every topic, every chapter, of this textbook.

It is important that a definition of communication disorder be provided. We have used a definition suggested by Van Riper requiring that the communication skills of an individual must be sufficiently different to (1) call negative attention, (2) interfere with communication, and/or (3) cause the speaker to be concerned.

There may be 23–24 million persons in the United States with some form of communication disorder. This figure demonstrates a clear need for specialists who are highly skilled in providing services to the communicatively impaired.

The study of speech/language pathology and audiology encompasses the several sciences from which a helping profession can develop. The practice of this profession, as of many others, involves the application of an art based on scientific knowledge. We hope this book clearly reflects the nature of the profession and its value to the communi-catively impaired.

SUGGESTED READINGS

Boone, D. R. (1987). *Human Communication and Its Disorders.* Englewood Cliffs, NJ: Pren-tice-Hall. *A thorough and objective introductory and survey textbook. It has an excel-lent review of scientific bases as well as a humanitarian sensitivity.*

Note: A number of "survey" books are available, each with special attractive features. Some are more "scientific," some emphasize certain disorders, some focus on age groups (e.g., children), but all are worth examining at a library.

Perkins, W. H. (1978). *Human Perspectives in Speech and Language Disorders.* St. Louis: C. V. Mosby. *A most readable and interesting presentation built around stories of real people, with objective information woven into the personal descriptions. The book covers all the speech and language disorders, but not hearing problems.*

Van Riper, C. (1978). *Speech Correction. Principles and Practices,* Englewood Cliffs, N.J.: Prentice-Hall. 6th ed. *Throughout its many editions this has been the most influential introductory text in the field. Many professionals owe their entry into the field to this sensitive and thorough coverage of the disorders. This or any edition will serve to fascinate the reader and demonstrate the human qualities of the author.*

Study Questions

1. Identify physical "differences" among your acquaintances. Examine eye color, body height, shape of nose, etc. In what ways are these differences important (*a*) to the person and (*b*) to you?

2. Do any of the differences you might find in acquaintances have significant effects on those persons? Are these effects handicapping?

3. Consider an anatomic difference in a person. Is it a defect? Is it handicapping?

4. What fields of work require normal hearing? Would you consider it discriminatory if you were to apply to enter one of those fields and were rejected because you had a hearing disorder?

5. How do "human" attitudes toward physical defects compare with "primitive" (e.g., animal packs or isolated forest tribes) attitudes? Do such attitudes differ in kind or degree (or both)?

6. How would your appraisal of yourself differ were you to have (*a*) a painful cut on your index finger, (*b*) loss of a thumb, (*c*) a wart on your nose, (*d*) loss of your tongue, (*e*) a weak heart, (*f*) a seriously defective heart?

7. Do you think that a person who stutters is not of normal intelligence? That a man who does not respond to his wife's conversation has a hearing impairment? That a woman who forgets her husband's name has a brain injury? Do you think some people answer "yes" to all of these?

8. Define "handicap," "disorder," "defect," "anomaly," "difference"; use two or more dictionaries.

2

Children's Language Development and Disorders

In this chapter we delve first into an overview of language and its major components. A general outline is given of the requirements a child must meet (the prerequisite capacities) for language learning; in a child who may not have learned language normally, one must probe these capacities for causal relationships. We then examine the steps a child might take when learning to use language; since these stages may be very generally associated with age, among other attributes of the child, chronologic development of language is examined.

Having a cursory understanding of some of the normal aspects of language learning, we next explore children's language disorders as a difference or deviation from what we consider normal. The somewhat specific characteristics of such disorders of communication are outlined. The remediation of children's language disorders is impossible to summarize. Considering the necessary prerequisites, the varied characteristics, and the distinction between primary and secondary disorders, one would find extremely wide-ranging variation in remediation programs. These programs are often individually structured and managed.

LANGUAGE AND LANGUAGE DEVELOPMENT

People communicate with each other by sharing thoughts, ideas, and feelings. Oral communication expresses these concepts by utilizing vocal sounds that groups of people have tacitly agreed to use in a common manner. This is oral language. A spoken language consists of those sounds to which meaning has been ascribed by a group of people. Different groups may use a variety of vocal sounds to express the same

9

thought, of course. However, a single principle occurs throughout all language groups: there is an agreed-upon set of vocalizations to which meaning has been assigned by common agreement.

A person moving from one language group to another without learning the second language may have a communication disorder of a type. The person neither understands the meaningful sounds vocalized by those in the second group nor uses their standard oral symbols for expressing feelings or ideas. Other pertinent examples are those children who for some reason have not learned to understand or to speak the language of the people around them. Moving to an older age group, another example is adults who, because of a brain injury, lose the ability to understand and speak the language they have always used and that is employed by those about them. Each illustration is an important language disorder.

A child usually learns a language over the period of a few years upon immersion in an oral language environment. What are the necessary ingredients in developing such a sophisticated and complex skill? We must look at the nature of both language itself and the child who learns to use it. We should acknowledge the influence of other stimuli such as other persons, visual impressions, auditory input, and so on.

Language is one means of communication. We communicate through a number of avenues. We use gestures, especially when we use a common gesture system such as signing and finger spelling, as is so well utilized with deaf persons. We write or draw pictures or point to illustrations to express an idea. Like other forms of animal life, we utter calls or vocal sounds of various types to indicate our position or our intentions. These alternative means of communication may be important, especially to persons (such as the deaf) who find oral language use difficult or limited.

THE NATURE OF LANGUAGE

A helpful definition of language by Lahey (see Suggested Readings) suggests it to be "a code whereby ideas about the world are represented through a conventional system of arbitrary signals for communication." Signals are words and sentences that are vocally produced. The vocal sounds that people use in talking with each other have been standardized within a language. A common vocalization of a specific sound combination is said to mean a particular thing; it is a meaningful word. These sounds are organized into words that are presented in orderly sequences (e.g., sentences) that are generally recognized by others familiar with that language. The sounds and words and sentences are used to serve the intentions of the speaker. The dimensions of oral language are *content, form,* and *use* (Fig. 2.1).

Content

We know that words represent things, or activities. Words are symbols. The study of word meaning is known as *semantics.* It is the content of language. A field of study in itself, filled with ramifications far beyond the simple level of vocabulary, semantics is an important aspect of language. Spoken words stand for something. The speaker must use specific words to mean a particular thing. A book cannot be called a

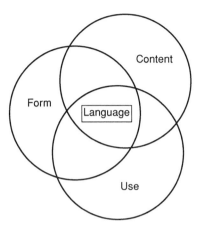

Figure 2.1. Dimensions of Normal Oral Language
Adapted from Lahey, M. (1988). *Language Disorders and Language Development.* New York: Macmillan.

tree. But the word "book" is not the thing "book." The word "book" stands for, or symbolizes, the thing. One cannot overgeneralize; one cannot call all printed material "books," just as one cannot call all animals or even all dogs "Bowser."

As content refers to the topic of expression, the meaning or the semantic aspect, it takes words to form that expression. This is vocabulary or lexicon. The two travel together, of course. One needs words to express the meanings one has. You might expect, or perhaps hope, that the more you have to say (the more ideas you have) the greater the number of words, and the more precise the vocabulary becomes.

> Children must acquire a vocabulary to gain the use of a large number of words to express ideas. They need to learn that the vocal sounds other people utter have meaning. Children must learn to process ideas and feelings using words, and need to learn to use those vocal sounds as words to tell other people what they are thinking about. Adults do this rather routinely, but some persons develop problems in semantic aspects. Forgetting a word, or not having the proper word at the proper time, or failing to understand a common word another person uses are examples of communication problems. One could say these are content-based language problems.

Form

A second aspect of language is the more structured dimension. This deals with the rule-directed grammar of the language, whether it is English or French or Turkish. Form consists of three subdimensions: syntax, phonology, and morphology.

Syntax refers to the sequential organization of words according to their relationships to each other. For example, the syntax of English requires that the order in which words are uttered cannot be changed very much, while in other languages word order may not be as important to express the same message.

If one wanted to indicate that a boy consumes a fruit, one might say "Boy ate apple," with possibly some descriptive words added that might change the meaning little. The English syntax rules forbid any other word order. For example, to send the message one cannot say "Apple ate boy" or, worse, "Ate boy apple."

Syntax adds to lexical meaning. It adds the component of relationship among words. In the preceding example, "Boy ate apple," the conjoining of the three words in their particular (rule-bound) order sums to more than the meaning of each of the words alone. As the old saying goes, the whole is greater than the sum of the parts.

Phonology is the use of the speech-sounds of the language. This, too, is rule-bound in each separate language. The speech-sounds are the phonemes (vowels and consonants) as well as the stress (vocal emphasis) and the intonation (melody). The first, phonemes, are sometimes referred to as the *segments* of the language, while the second is often termed the *suprasegmental* component. The rule aspect states that we are limited in our language as to how we combine phonemes: e.g., "fmoorl" is unacceptable.

In the next chapter, the production of the segments will be discussed under the label *articulation*. This is an older term, slowly being subsumed under phonology. A definite relationship is intended between the two, but in the present material, the distinction refers to phoneme rules and to the vocal emphasis (stress) and change in pitch (intonation). This is different from the formation of the speech-sounds in the oral cavity by the vocal tract, aspects of oral communication that will be discussed later.

Morphology refers to the use of morphemes, the smallest units of language (not speech) that carry meaning. Remember that a phoneme is a vowel or consonant that need not carry meaning in itself; a morpheme is required to carry meaning. These linguistic structural units are of two kinds. One can stand alone and carry content in doing so. Words such as "dog" or "milk" or "Daddy" carry content; these are meaningful morphemes. The other type of morpheme must be bound to a free-standing morpheme to be meaningful. It adds an additional meaning component. To the preceding examples, which are able to stand alone, we may add bound morphemes. We can change the meaning of "dog" by adding *s,* thus producing a plural word that has more meaning than "dog" alone. We can change the word "milk" to "milked" and completely change the word and its meaning. And, we can change the word "Daddy" to "Daddy's," adding a possessive character and thereby changing the original word. So, morphologic changes allow us to add a dimension of time, of number, and of possession, among other intentions.

Use

The use to which language is put is pragmatics. This suggests the purposes of speaking. The intention of the speaker is clarified by the way language is expressed. Pragmatics is a dimension beyond the selection of the proper words or placing them in meaningful order. Pragmatics also considers the particular situation, the environment, and the social context in which the speaker is talking. It takes into consideration what the listener should know about the utterance and its context.

When an utterance is not comprehended, this could occur because the listener was not "cued in." Although the order in which the speaker placed sounds and words might have been correct according to form and content criteria, it was not understood because the speaker did not utilize a context in which the listener could place what was said; the listener did not grasp the speaker's intention. What was said was ambiguous. It was not what the speaker "meant."

What might be intended when your companion states, "The speed limit in this state is 55 miles per hour"? You will probably answer: "It depends." It depends on the situation and what your companion knows about you. If you are walking together along a street, it could mean one thing. If you are sitting in traffic court, it could mean something else. If your companion is a passenger in the car you are driving, it could have other meanings. To complicate the matter, your companion could make the statement a question, or an emotional statement, a scream, or a flat and discouraged muttering. The form in which your companion makes the statement expresses the intention as well as the words themselves. Language use, then, is a complex process requiring skill not only in using words and phrases, but in placing them in a context that accurately indicates your intentions.

Of course, spoken language does not just appear. It develops. Child language development occurs in a youngster who is capable of developing language. What are the capacities, the prerequisites, children must have in order to learn the language spoken around them?

PREREQUISITE CAPACITIES FOR LANGUAGE LEARNING

Human beings as biologic creatures are classified in the animal kingdom. Much of the nature of humans is similar to that of many animals that are not human. This is especially true of our anatomies and physiologic systems. But with the development of language usage, of vocal speech, through the functioning of a unique brain, the human animal became the talking human being. Humans had some certain special capacities for this behavior organized in such a way that only they could learn to talk as they did. Children must have those capacities as well (Fig. 2.2).

First, children must have something to say, of course, to learn to talk. They must have ideas, or feelings, or notions about themselves and how they tie in with the world and people around them. They must think. They must have some *intellectual* capacity. Intelligence suggests learning, perceiving, understanding, concept processing, appropriate responding. Intellectual capacity refers to the child's ability to learn and especially to learn language. Intelligence, or cognition, is exemplified by the ability to identify objects and events, to understand them, to differentiate among them, and to function appropriately. The learning from these activities causes appropriate behavioral changes. The intellectual capacity becomes the comparator against which language use is balanced.

It is not difficult to illustrate the lack of intellectual skills in language learning by pointing to children variously identified as mentally retarded. Observing the effect of diminished cognitive capacity, one notes their language usage (from vocabulary through syntax to pragmatic aspects) to be similar to that of younger children. Chronologic age leads to certain expectations. Mental age, however, is the determiner for the the child's language level. A child who has just observed his/her fifth birthday, for example, but whose mental age (by some testing procedure) is three years will probably have the language abilities of a three-year-old child.

The second capacity necessary to develop language is that of *sensory-perceptual* abilities. This cannot be completely divorced from intelligence, for the two may have a close interrelationship. It is important, however, to point to the sensory and the perceptual capacities, for these are primary input modalities for language learning.

The *sensory* component of this capacity indicates the importance of being aware of one's environment. It refers more importantly to audition, the ability to hear the language being spoken in the environment. The child's hearing sense picks up the spoken language from the society; the brain perceives it by "making sense" of the spoken words and associating it to experience. A record is made in the child's memory.

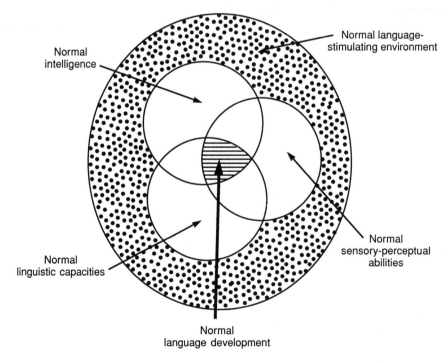

Figure 2.2. The Capacities for Normal Language Development
Adapted from Lahey, M. (1988). *Language Disorders and Language Development.* New York: Macmillan.

As the child continues to hear others talking, he/she practices talking. Children learn to speak the language spoken around them. A child in an English-speaking home and environment will not learn German or Swahili, but will learn English, of course. What is heard and perceived is what is spoken.

An example of sensory deprivation can be found in auditory sensation. Illustrative is the child born without hearing. A deaf child may have serious difficulties learning to talk. The sophistication of expanding vocabulary, of forming grammatically complex sentences, of developing skill in using language is a complex task for the deaf child. When special efforts are not made to assist such children, then speech and language may be extremely limited. Auditory sensory deficit can be a serious detriment to a child's language learning.

The *perceptual* component refers to the child's ability to receive and recognize stimuli (such as hearing speech). To perceive something is to be aware or conscious of it, to have knowledge of it, to discriminate it from other events or conditions, and to retain that information. Infants are aware of and respond to the sound of their mother's voice as opposed to other person's voices; they can distinguish between and among words, even vowel sounds, although they have not learned to utter them yet. This perceptual process seems to develop before oral expression is used, although the nature of the process is not entirely clear.

A third prerequisite to the child's learning to talk is *linguistic capacity.* This suggests that the human being has an inborn system for language processing, for language learning. It represents a "potential" for language use, a capability that requires stimulation to function. Simply stated, there is a built-in system that is ready to be put to use in processing and programming language. Having a system and using it may be two different things.

A fourth capacity for normal language development in a child is the *neurologic system.* To the earlier noted sensory capacity one must add the other neurologic systems, including that component associated with muscle actions. One learns by doing. The child follows a language model, which is spoken all around, by patterning muscle activities to say the same things he/she hears.

A fifth capacity deals with the *emotional component.* A personality responsive to other people and to linguistic stimuli is important to language development. Whether emotions are isolated characteristics or stem from physiologic mechanisms (such as hormones or other biochemical mechanisms) is not germane at this point, but certainly emotional stability may be related to those variables.

Lastly, language development is dependent upon an *environment* that is linguistic. Children learn the language they hear. The model that is set before them and the happy consequences of following that model, in learning to talk, are very important to normal language development.

Inborn linguistic capacity can be compared with a similar programmed ability of the human to walk on two, not four, feet. Anatomically (including physiologically and neurologically), we are born with the potential for bipedal locomotion. We need to be placed in a situation in which we learn to walk that way. Similarly, we are born with the capability to *learn* to talk (note the emphasis). We must put to use that capability.

There is an interdependence among these capacities. Associating meaning to verbal signals is a language or symbolic task. It requires intellectual capacity, sensory-perceptual capacity, linguistic capacity, and more. Carrying out the symbolic task (using or manipulating linguistic symbols) involves concepts. Retention and modification of concepts are based, to some extent, upon feedback loops, events (internal and external) responding to the language processing that influence the concept of the linguistic task. Some external input and feedback events are found in the child's environment.

Other prerequisites related to the development of language in the child include a *language-stimulating environment.* This indicates that communicative efforts by the child are supported by adults who not only are caring but are responsive to those efforts. A "talking" environment triggers the capacities to language use. One more prerequisite, or capacity, that modern researchers are investigating is motor speech processing. The brain's ability to plan and then to sequence the necessary movements to produce speech and language is considered by some to be an essential inborn capability.

In summary, it seems safe to say that the child will learn to talk using the language spoken in his/her environment if at least four capacities and prerequisites are intact and interactive. That is, the child must have reasonably normal intellectual skills, sensory-perceptual abilities, and linguistic programming built into a language-learning and language-producing system. The mutual interdependence of these capacities on each other needs further study and exploration, especially in remedial situations.

It is important to point out that the child's capacities must be stimulated by talking people in his/her environment, the language-stimulating talking world. Without input, there is limited output. We are speaking here of an average, normal child with average or normal audition, average or normal perceptual abilities, average or normal intellectual capacities, and lastly, a programmed language system ready to be set into operation.

STAGES OF LANGUAGE DEVELOPMENT

All children do not develop in the same way at the same rate. For example, it is far from true that all one-year-old children can walk, turn around, and stand on one foot. Perhaps some can. Perhaps some can just barely elevate themselves to a standing position, let alone cover some distance walking. Similar statements can probably be made concerning such skills as toilet training or self-feeding or talking. Of course it is important to believe that a child is developing "on schedule"; but the schedule for normal developmental skill acquisition has some normal variation. We start with the notion of some rather distinct steps or stages of development. Then we associate those skill levels with age *ranges,* not specific chronologic (years and months) age. We can associate a number of developmental changes with chronologic age, usually expecting the variation in age level to agree with the child's chronologic age (Fig. 2.3).

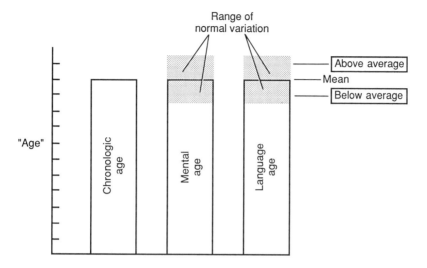

Figure 2.3.   Ranges of "Age" Scores Compared with Chronologic Age
Note: Chronologic age is not a score but a counting of months/years since birth. The scores are measures on tests. Normal is a *range* around a mean. The statistical mean should match chronologic age.

A two-sided measurement is made. One is the measurement of the age range, the other is the measurement of language acquisition. The first is not difficult. The second is somewhat more complicated than counting months and years. When assessing language, what does one "count"? What are the measured "scores"?

One approach is to count the number of words a child uses. Were you to be asked to do this, how would you go about it? Would you listen to the child, clicking a counter for each word uttered? How long would you have to do this? A minute? An hour? Longer? You probably could devise a number of objections to such a measurement. Rather than an overall count, perhaps you could create some sort of an average. You might count the number of words the child uses on the average every five minutes, or ten minutes. One could imagine the variation that might occur.

One common approach is to count the average number of words the child uses each time he/she speaks. To objectify it further, morphemes (see earlier definition) are counted to develop a mean or average. This average is called the *mean length of utterance* (MLU). Ideally, 100 talking events are evaluated for the number of morphemes in each utterance; an average or mean is easily computed from these data. The MLU has provided a way of establishing stages of development. Tables 2.1, 2.2, and 2.3 present developmental information with increasing details. Table 2.1 provides five major stages with appropriate MLUs. Table 2.2 increases the detail, adding substages, ranges of MLU for various stages, and the predicted or chronologic ages for each substage. Finally, Table 2.3 completes the description by providing the development of linguistic skills beyond the MLU for each stage.

Table 2.1.   Mean Length of Utterance Stages (Brown)

STAGE	MLU (MIDPOINT OF RANGE)
1	1.75
2	2.25
3	2.75
4	3.75
5	4.50

Adapted from Brown, R. (1973). *A First Language: The Early Stages.* Cambridge, MA: Harvard University Press.

Table 2.2.   Brown's Stages of Language Development

STAGE	MLU RANGE	PREDICTED AGE RANGE (MONTHS)[a]
Early stage I	1.01–1.49	16.4–27.5
Late stage I	1.50–1.99	19.3–32.3
Stage II	2.00–2.49	22.3–37.7
Stage III	2.50–2.99	24.7–41.6
Early stage IV	3.00–3.49	28.8–46.6
Late stage IV–early stage V	3.50–3.99	31.6–48.5
Late stage V	4.00–4.49	37.5–52.9
Post-stage V	4.50–6.00	41.0–66.7

Adapted from Miller, J. F. (1981). *Assessing Language Production in Children.* Baltimore: University Park Press.
[a] The correlation between age in months and mean length of response; Brown's stages are subdivided, and predicted age ranges include one standard deviation above and below the mean to include 68% of the population studied.

Table 2.3.   Language Development from 1.0 Morphemes to 4.5 Morphemes

The ages at which these particular aspects of language development occur are variant. The order of development and the changes that occur at each "stage," which is determined by MLU, are quite invariant, not only across children but even across languages. Often, each stage is further subdivided (e.g., "early" or "late").

Stage I.   **Semantic Roles and Grammatical Relations**
Covers an MLU between 1.0 and 2.0 morphemes.
Age range: 16–31 months.
One, two, and three word utterances.
Semantic relations: agent-action, action-object, action-locative, entity-locative, entity-attribute, demonstrative-entity.
Yes-no questions signaled by rising intonation; e.g., "See kitty?"
Limited set of *wh*-questions.

Stage II. **Grammatical Morphemes and the Modulation of Meaning**

Covers an MLU between 2.0 and 2.5 morphemes.

Age range: 21–35 months.

Addition of grammatical morphemes, tense markers, plurals, articles, possessive markers, auxiliaries, the copula, third-person regular, and the prepositions *in* and *on*; usually not heard 100% of the time until the child is past
stage V.

Negative elements.

Stage III. **Modalities of the Simple Sentence**

Covers an MLU between 2.5 and 3.0 morphemes.

Age range: 24–41 months.

Length increases mainly the result of the auxiliary, which enables the child
to make interrogative and negative sentences more closely resembling the
adult form.

Increase in the number of *wh*-questions.

Interrogative reversals.

Polite phrases; e.g., "Please," "Thank you." *Because* appears.

Stage IV. **Embedding**

Covers an MLU between 3.0 and 3.5 morphemes.

Age range: 28–50 months.

Major linguistic change that increases length at this stage is the embedding
of one sentence into a semantic role of another sentence; e.g., (1) object-
noun-phrase complements, such as "We know, we just do it to ya"; (2) in-
direct or embedded *wh*-questions, such as "I don't know what I ate"; (3)
relative clauses, such as "Here ones that don't belong here." Begins *aren't,
doesn't,* as well as *how* and *when,* etc.

Stage V. **Coordination of Simple Sentences and Propositional Relations**

Covers an MLU between 3.5 and 4.5 morphemes.

Age range: 37–52 + months.

Coordination of two simple sentences; e.g., "He hit me right here and it
hurt."

Coordination of two sentences with deletion; e.g., "My mommy and daddy
don't eat candy."

Locatives; e.g., *up, down*; indefinites (*nobody, none, nothing*) added. . . .

Main conjunction is *and*, but *if* and *because*, etc., come into use. . . .

Adapted from Brown, R. (1978). *A First Language: The Early Stages.* Cambridge, MA: Harvard University Press.

There are a number of problems in measuring language development by using
the mean length of utterance. Remember that in counting morphemes, one counts
words and meaningful added components. If a child of 18 months, in an appropriate
situation, utters "Daddy dinner," does he/she mean "Daddy eats dinner," or "That's
Daddy's dinner," or "Get Daddy's dinner"? The intention of the utterance may remain
uncertain. Suppose the child states "Daddy's dinner." Excluding the possibility that

the child means that Daddy is the entree for dinner, the best guess might be that the plate on the table contains food belonging to his/her father. By adding one element, the *s,* the meaning is enhanced. One must count the word with such an addition when measuring language development.

By adding the *s* to his/her choice of words, the 18-month-old in the example also could provid another grammatical component to his/her language skill. This child could add the concept of *possession:* the dinner belongs to Daddy. Possessiveness is one aspect of language *maturation.*

Another aspect to be learned relates to *tense,* to time. Early in development, the child learns about present, past, and future. Just learning that some occurrences take place in other than the present time is a step forward. Learning about yesterday and tomorrow is an additional refinement to the child's language skill.

Yet another development in the use of language occurs when children learn to talk about what is not visibly present in their environment. At first a child speaks about what is visible in the immediate surroundings, the "here and now." That is a hard enough step to take, to find appropriate morphemes for those things or events that impinge upon the child's senses at that moment. A more difficult step is for the child to talk about something that is out of sight, or past in time, or yet to happen. All three of these are at different levels of complexity. The idea of *object permanence,* the symbolic representation of something when it is not present, is an important acquisition in learning to use language meaningfully.

Lastly, *language comprehension* abilities as they emerge in the developing child are critical to the totality of what is called "language learning." This refers to the child's skill to grasp the meaning of spoken language. So far, limited research efforts have been made to better understand the language comprehension of children. Language production has been vigorously studied, as is evident in the preceding pages. Studying language comprehension is a complex activity. More than likely, it will become an important aspect of child study as well as a major component in evaluating language development.

CHRONOLOGIC DEVELOPMENT OF LANGUAGE USE

Nearly everyone seems to appreciate associating an age with an event. We start this early in our lives by identifying a month and day with a birthdate and other important events and holidays in our lives. We associate certain age levels with other events, such as an age at which we can vote, or drive a car, or retire, or engage in other activities. And we expect to hear reports about children as to their development, quickly comparing that developmental level with some imagined standard of normalcy or brilliance.

We expect children to be talking at increasingly complex levels with increasing age. It is, however, an error for us to be very specific about the age in months at which a child should be speaking in certain skilled ways. If on his/her first birthday the youngster is not speaking words (or phrases or sentences or paragraphs), there is some danger that an observer might consider the child to be less than normal. The observer's definition of "normal" hinges upon an impression of what is supposed to be evident on a certain date in a certain time of life, such as the first birthday. We are much wiser to speak of chronologic development of language skills in terms of ranges, not in specific months. It is true, of course, that we continue to associate age with developmental skill acquisition. But, we usually define the level as an age range; that is, the child should have developed a certain skill between the ages of six and eight months, or four and five years, or at six years plus-or-minus 18 months.

With such a warning or caveat, it might be safe to place some landmarks in language development into a chronologic framework. Whatever the boundaries of an age range might be, one should keep in mind that there is some overlap between stages. If the age range being discussed is, for example, between 18 and 24 months, nothing magical happens at the 18th month or the 24th month point, for these "points" also are a part of a range. The development is continuous, not jumping from age range to age range.

At the outset, the youngster uses the vocal tract to produce a variety of sounds and noises, initiated by the nervous system, stimulated and modeled by the child's awareness of other people's vocal sounds and noises as they communicate around him/her. The social bonding taking place is reflected in part by the child's participation. The sensory-perceptual capacity functions early, perhaps within a month of birth if not before. Infants are able to discriminate between some vowel sounds, suggesting they have an intact sensory-perceptual capacity. The infant in the first six months of life develops the ability to recognize other aspects of phonologic development: he/she can tell the difference between sounds when the difference is in manner of articulation, or in place of articulation, or in voicing. The child establishes a feature (Chapter 3) analysis system extremely early in life. This partially supports the theory that there is an inborn linguistic capacity that is ready to be programmed by language stimulation from other people.

During the first few months, the child is also producing communicative acts with his/her unskilled language system (Table 2.4). At first such acts revolve around very

---

Table 2.4. Normal Prelinguistic Vocalizations and Onset of Speech

---

Early vocalizations of normally developing infants progress through a sequence of four broad stages. These will be briefly described with approximate ages of onset; it should be remembered, however, that there is considerable individual variation regarding age of occurrence.

Stage I.   In the first few months of life, the great majority of vocalizations can be described as discomfort (crying, fussing) or as vegetative (coughing, burping, etc.) sounds that have little in common with the sounds in the production of speech.

Stage II.   About the end of the second month, the infant begins to produce vocalizations typically referred to as "coos" or "goos." Acoustically, these utterances are similar to back vowels (e.g., /u/) or syllables consisting of back consonants (e.g., /k/, /g/) followed by back vowels. As Oller (1980)[a] points out, the consonant-vowel combinations produced at this stage should be considered "primitive" syllables since the timing of opening and closure of the consonantal and vocalic elements is far less regular than that observed in adult speech.

Stage III.   Between 7 and 9 months of age, infants begin to produce vocalizations that are increasingly speechlike. The utterances are typically longer and consist of well-defined consonant-vowel syllables much like those of adult speech. The striking characteristic of the productions at this stage is the presence of reduplicated consonant-vowel sequences, e.g., /mamama/, /dididi/. Upon hearing a sequence such as /mama/ or /dada/, parents often report with delight that their 7-month-old child has begun to call them by name. At this stage of development, however, there is no evidence of denotative meaning associated with the sounds produced.

Stage IV.   Toward the end of the first year, usually around 10–11 months, infants begin to produce "variegated" babbling. The vocalizations that characterize this stage are similar to those of the preceding period in that they, too, consist of sequences of consonant-vowel syllables. The reduplicative nature of the syllables is no longer present, however, and a variety of consonants or vowels can co-occur in a single utterance, e.g., /bawidu/. A second characteristic of this stage is the presence of intonational patterns similar to those of the adult language the infant is learning. Many parents report they feel their child is producing whole sentences—statements, questions, exclamations—but in their "own language." Stage IV is followed closely by the emergence of recognizable words, usually around 13–15 months of age. The syllabic structure and the sounds of these words are often similar to those which occur in the late babbling stage, but for the first time the sequence of sounds is consistently paired with a meaning and is identifiable as an attempt at an adult word.

From Stoel-Gammon, C. (1981). Speech development of infants and children with Down's syndrome. Chapter 15 in *Speech Evaluation in Medicine*, J. K. Darby, Ed., pp. 341–360. New York: Grune & Stratton.
[a] Reference provided in Stoel-Gammon (1981).

basic behaviors such as cries, or laughter, or sucking. This skill continues to the third month to be refined into infantile behaviors such as cooing and then babbling. This last activity approaches speech-sound productions, although rarely with precision or consistency. Up to the ninth month, when a speech-sound is produced and proves to be satisfying to the child in some way, it may be repeated. Chains of repeated speech-sounds often occur as the child learns to talk.

Jimmie, at age four months, often followed the completion of drinking a nursing bottle of milk with some "talking," perhaps more to himself than to anyone else. His lips would meet with great satisfaction as he voiced different kinds of sounds. So, he could be heard repeating: "ma-ma-ma" or "ba-ba-ba" or perhaps even "da-da-da." Sometimes a chortle of delight followed or accompanied his babbling. On the other hand, down the street was little Les who was much less vigorous and active in many things, including babbling. After nursing, Les occasionally could be heard vocalizing but not babbling. He did not seem to enjoy the act of making the noises so very much akin to the speech-sounds used by adults in his environment. In fact, at four months Les was just beginning to be aware of individuals' voices, so that he would turn to the sound of his mother's voice but not utter anything in particular in response. The question arises, then, is Les delayed in development or is Jimmie precocious, or are they both within the *range* of normalcy? Perhaps this is a question that can be answered only at a later age or developmental level.

Toward the end of the second six months there is an increase of vocal activities and recognition of linguistic activities of other persons in the environment. Part of this period is labeled by some language specialists as the "prelinguistic" stage; others consider it truly "linguistic," if only because more receptive and perceptive skills in language use are developing in the child. The youngster now begins to understand speech patterns, such as those of anger or those in praise. He/she responds, to indicate understanding. When mother forcefully pronounces "No" as the child reaches for an extension cord or other potentially dangerous object, the reaction of withdrawal and then cries of fear or upset follow to signal not only understanding of the utterance but an opinion of that denial.

The average child in this second half of the first year will begin using syllables, blending consonants with vowels. The strings of such utterances are duplicated frequently. Some of these come very close to words, and in fact may be just that. Phonologic (articulation) development also is moving along. Some tongue-tip sounds are added to the already established tongue-back sounds; more sounds using the lips appear. An intonation pattern is beginning, similar to that which the child hears.

Great pride ensues when a youngster's first word is uttered. The father of little Kris was ecstatic when as he entered her room, she smiled at him from her crib and said "Da-da, da-da." This was obviously (according to him) her first word. The fact that it could be interpreted as her acknowledgment of his paternity biases the observation considerably, of course. Yet it is difficult to deny him the satisfaction, or her the credit. On the other hand, Nickie (on hearing her father enter her room) might cry aloud, obviously unaccepting of the role her father played. Both children being somewhat over nine months of age, the differences in their use of "language" would be apparent, and would receive responses of differing types as well. Such responses can act to encourage or discourage, to reward or punish, to stimulate additional efforts or fail to so stimulate them. The building of a supportive communicative framework in that social situation is one of the beginnings of social language skill.

At about one year, the child should be approaching regular use of single words; perhaps the first word will be heard in the vicinity of the first birthday—but even that as a definite and specific "point" of age should be avoided. It is only an approximation of the age range in which the first word should become a regular aspect of the youngster's ability to talk. This age range, in and about the first birthday, is uncertain in its boundaries. Some specialists place it between nine and 18 months, while others narrow the range to between 12 and 18 months. Table 2.4 indicates that the first recognizable words usually occur between 13 and 15 months.

Here, and elsewhere in the developmental sequencing, the youngster increases his/her use of language. The pragmatic component becomes more sophisticated. The step-by-step sequence is yet to be quantified, but some generalities do occur. The "use" aspect will be noted here, but is little discussed elsewhere because of the scarcity of factual information. We note, for example, such linguistic behaviors as underinclusion, in which a word has only one referent, not a generic one. The word "dog" may mean only the child's dog but not all dogs. On the other hand, overinclusion refers to the use of the word "dog" to mean dogs as well as cats and other animals.

Following the 12th month and up to the 18th month, the youngster's language skills increase. Perceptually, the child increases his/her recognition vocabulary to a great extent. Perceptual skills become more complex. Word relationships, such as "Mommy's car" or "Doggie's food" are recognized. The youngster demonstrates increased pragmatic sophistication in productive abilities. He/she talks more about the surrounding world. The child sees an object on the floor and loudly proclaims it as "Mommy shoe," or sees his/her drink on the table and indicates "Drink milk." Phonologic skills increase; additional phonemes are produced, although inconsistencies as well as gaps in yet-to-be-acquired speech-sound vocabulary are common.

> Merry was born with Down syndrome, a genetic defect associated with mental retardation among other effects. Her apparent awareness of her immediate environment remained her primary focus for many months. At 18 months, and still at two years, and even in later months and years, she was more interested in what she could see, hear, touch, or otherwise sense than in what was not present. Merry remained more concerned about the clothes she had on at the moment, a trivial bump on her hand, the sound of a dog barking at the moment, flashing lights, or other immediate stimuli. The concept of verb tenses or even of some possessives would be difficult for Merry. Her language skill development was obviously delayed.

Toward the end of this period, as the child approaches 18 months object permanency develops. The child is no longer bound to talk about, or consider, just what is in sight. He/she does not have to talk about the "here and now," but can go beyond, and can refer to what is out of sight, what is not "here." No longer is "out of sight, out of mind" true. The child observes the lack of objects, as well as the presence of them. For example, he/she might note: "No doggie," when there is reason to think an animal might be present, or looking at the dinner table might observe that someone is lacking and proclaim: "Daddy gone." Such perceptual development offers a basis for greatly expanded language use, the ability to talk in the abstract and to consider more than concrete and observable objects. One might associate this with memory, or recall; this is closely tied to intellectual capacity.

Approaching the 24th month, and entering the "terrible twos," the young-ster's perceptual abilities continue to advance. He/she now is aware of spoken direc-tions or commands and can follow a single-order command. The child may obey when asked: "Find your truck," or "Bring your ball with you." Some definite and profitable relationship occurs in such commands. The youngster not only has grasped object permanence (e.g., where the truck or the ball is, even if out of sight), but realizes that retrieving the object accompanies another activity yet to take place. All of this represents highly abstract cognitive ability.

Both perceptual and productive abilities allow the child to grasp two-word relationships. Perceptually, for example, he/she understands that the object on the chair is "Daddy's hat" or that the toy on the floor is the "big truck" (not a smaller one elsewhere). As one result of this perceptual skill development, the youngster now is heard making two-word utterances. Certainly by the second birthday, if not before, the child should provide two words meaningfully in a noun-plus-verb sentence: "Mommy go," "Baby eat," and so on. The phonologic skills continue to be enhanced so that a child in this age range should produce both voiced and unvoiced speech-sound pairs fairly readily. Differentiating between conditions of phonation in speaking is a hall-mark of development here.

Probably one of the most fascinating and perhaps irritating language behaviors (to some associates of two-year-olds) is the development of the question. The *"wh-"* questions start. Parents find themselves answering "Why?" more frequently than they find comfortable. More than likely, however, it is only an indication of the more sophisticated and complex behavior that is developing in the child.

As the child develops sophistication, **moving toward the 30-month age range,** we find increased perceptual abilities developing. The child can understand pronouns and knows "he" and "she." At the same time, perhaps because of that magic of the second year of life, the youngster begins to understand negative sentences (perhaps because so many are uttered in his/her presence). "Do not do that!" should be understood by this time. The child is also refining an understanding of others' questions. He/she can grasp the meaning of more complex questions, including those about objects that are out of sight. Productively, the talking behavior of the 2½-year-old should include a simple sentence. It might be a two-word or a three-word sentence, but it should be a noun- or verb-phrase, however simple it might be. Phonologically, the youngster adds new types of speech-sounds to his/her phonetic vocabulary.

Bill, at age 2½ years, had wedged himself thoroughly into the activities of his family. Physically active, inquisitive, explorative, and questioning are all terms one might use to describe him. Others might say he was hyperactive, got into everything, played with the piano and the silverware and the tools on his father's workbench, and constantly badgered everyone with hundreds of questions. Unfortunately, he was extremely difficult to understand. His phonologic development (his acquisition of speech sounds) was such that what language skills he had were obscured by less than adequate speech-sound production. He had not developed phoneme mastery commensurate with his language skills. Someone said he "talked baby talk." With his invasive behavior, this problem in making himself understood increasingly upset him and his short temper often appeared. His family began to react; some ignored his demands or questions, others interpreted for him, others handed him whatever object was nearest. Obviously, this reaction to his communication attempt even further exacerbated the situation. Bill's expectations for himself, as well as his family's expectations for him, were not being met. A communication disorder had developed.

Growing older, **toward the 36-month age,** the child's perceptual abilities increase and refine. He/she recognizes prepositions and more negatives; modifiers of various types are understood. Appropriate, adultlike word-order relationships begin to occur. The youngster begins to grasp the notion of color concepts. Numbers, beyond the concept of plurality, may be understood as well. Both color and number have far to go, of course, but a beginning is usually observed by the third birthday.

Productively, the infamous "*wh-*" questions develop more intensely. We hear lots of questions "Why?" and "What?" and "Where?" "When?" is also initiated, for the idea of time is one the child can now grasp in its simplest form. He/she understands a little about the present and the past, if not the future. The three-year-old's language also shows knowledge of cause-and-effect relationships, as well as possession—that something belongs to someone. The youngster probably has some infinitives in his/her spoken language at this age as well.

Phonologically, the three-year-old should develop more speech-sounds. All the vowel sounds should be acquired. Many three-year-old form the sibilant consonants well (Chapter 3), such as the /s/ sound. Others do not have full acquisition of these sibilant sounds at this age; in fact, some do not develop full skill in /s/-sound production until the age of seven or even eight years.

Taking a look at the language development of the average **four-year-old** should uncover real advancement in perceptual skills. In this age range, the child should be able to understand and follow two-order commands rather routinely. A request to put on a coat and close the door would be understood (and perhaps obeyed) by most four-year-olds. In fact, the child's understanding of complex grammatical utterances by other people is developing well. Now, sentences with prepositional phrases are understood. The four-year-old has a solid grasp of negatives as heard in the language of people in the environment. A fairly good understanding of spoken language has been acquired by this age level, and at this stage the child can engage in a conversation—a real dialogue.

In language production, the four-year-old uses prepositions fairly well. Plurals are present, although there are some that could be troublesome. Possessives have already been in the child's vocabulary to some extent, but by this age range he/she should have common use of this grammatical form in everyday talking.

The four-year-old's phonologic development in everyday speech is one of refining already developed speech-sound skills. Consonant blends or clusters creep in and are welcome additions to conversational speech (see Chapter 3). The refinement stage, linguistically and phonologically, is marked during this fourth year not by dramatic acquisitions but rather by refinements and extended use throughout the youngster's talking.

This refinement process continues through the next year, up into the **60th month, the fifth year of age.** One could identify specific changes, of course, although they might classify as polishing or extending already developed abilities. For example, the youngster will now be able to extend his/her understanding of commands beyond the two-order command to the three-order command. The child should be able to obey correctly a parent's directions to wash his/her hands, bring a chair, and drink a cup of milk without too much confusion.

The child's perceptual skills expand further into concepts such as time: the meaning of today, yesterday, and tomorrow. The understanding of number concepts, including plurals, expands considerably by the fifth year of age. The youngster should know the colors very well, at least most of the basic ones that are reinforced in everyday living. The five-year-old's perceptual abilities should include spatial relationships, locating objects in the real world fairly accurately.

The five-year-old's linguistic understandings also are expanded. Sentences with two adjectives are grasped quite well. And, although aspects may have developed earlier, the child should now have a good knowledge of what is meant when questioned: how much, how far, when, and the like. Comprehension of form or syntactic relationships is maturing.

The expressive skills of the five-year-old also demonstrate more mature abilities. Fairly complex sentences are produced, embedding two ideas within a single sentence, for example. The child has added reflexive pronouns by this age, probably further exploring his/her place in the surrounding world. He/she asks questions beginning "How" and "Why" and "Which." The five-year-old's language use, or productive skill, is nearly adultlike.

The child's speech should be nearly completely intelligible. Many of the speech sounds of his/her language should have been acquired, with some few exceptions. Some sibilants remain difficult, depending upon their locus in words. Some consonant blends may remain inconsistently produced, perhaps appearing as "cute" pronunciation errors rather than phonologic ones.

The five-year-old child, then, should be capable of understanding almost any linguistic form. Of course there will be vocabulary problems, but then vocabulary-building is a life-long activity, not one reserved to children as they develop linguistic skills. The mature level that the youngster has reached opens many doors: the main one is school. Now, the child is capable of meeting the challenge of education. He/she has the basic tool—language—to provide the means of learning more and more. The child has had language before this age, to be sure, and has learned a great deal up to this age; now the five-year old should have sufficient and mature enough language skills to meet educational, social, and even personal testing. In kindergarten the average five-year-old's language skills will find full utilization as the child begins his/her educational experiences.

Jessie's mother took her to the nearby school in September to enroll the girl in kindergarten. The teacher made it a point to screen all new children individually, talking with them, showing them the classroom and objects therein, and getting to know the youngsters. In Jessie's screening, the teacher was unable to understand much of what the child said. She spoke in short "sentences" of two or three words, her words were quite unclear, and she failed to remember where the door to the room was or where her mother was. The teacher recommended to the mother that she should not enter the child into kindergarten, but should seek special language and speech help at a local speech and language clinic. The delay in speech and language development that Jessie seemed to have also delayed her total educational program.

Beyond the fifth year of normal language development, the child will continue to advance language skills. At or around five years of age, a simple conversation can take place. The child can understand most of what is said; comprehension has developed to a most useful level. But much remains to be learned, perhaps all through the remaining lifetime. Language use develops into writing and reading abilities. New rules of morphology, sophisticated pragmatic (use) dimensions, and a continuously developing lexicon (supply of vocabulary) are acquired through the growing and developing years. Going to college is in many ways seen as a language development enhancement activity. Perhaps one could describe "learning" as the same. Does it ever cease?

Summary of Language and Normal Language Development

We need some background in order to understand children's language disorders. First, it is important to know about language itself, to grasp its various aspects of content, form, and use. Second, we must know the nature of children and what specifically they need to develop language skills. They need three basic prerequisites: intellectual capacity, sensory-perceptual capacity, and linguistic capacity. They must be normally intact and healthy children living in a normal-speaking environment. Third, we should be aware that children proceed through developmental stages in learning language. Development indicates age ranges, not just months or years of a specific age point. When the language skills of a youngster are assessed, the examination must cover all three components. We may wish to add others to further expand our knowledge of the developing child. When language disorders are identified, how are they displayed? What types of language problems occur, and how do we go about handling them?

CHILDREN'S LANGUAGE DISORDERS

Children may have difficulty speaking the language used in their environment. Most of them develop words, expand their vocabularies, engage in acceptable grammatical expressions, and carry on conversations at the usual age levels or earlier. Other children, the ones discussed here, are slower in learning to use this complex skill. As you might expect, there is great variability among these youngsters in just how delayed they might be. Some are but a little late, and even then only in narrow or special aspects. Others can be rather severely delayed in developing language skills.

They can demonstrate problems in forms of communication other than speaking; reading and writing problems can accompany speaking problems.

Oral language problems are identified by a number of different terms. Each term is not always synonymous with all the others; some experts ascribe very special and separate meanings to some terms. At this introductory level (with some exceptions) the student might find discussions of this subject in other references under the titles: language learning disorders, specific language disorders, primary language disorders, childhood aphasia, severe language disorders, language impairment, and language handicaps, among others.

The label applied here, children's language disorders, is used so that we can study the phenomenon from the perspective of children and the capacities they need for language learning, as well as from the perspective of language and the dimensions we can assign to language. Remember that the capacities necessary for learning language are three: normal sensory-perceptual capacity, linguistic capacity, and cognitive capacity. These must occur in a stimulating social environment. The underlying reason for a child failing to develop oral language skills in the usual manner and at the expected age lies in one of these capacities. One must assume, of course, that the language is being spoken normally by other people somewhere in the child's environment. Figure 2.4 presents schemes illustrating the effect on language of diminished capacities or of environment.

Recall also that to study language disorders, one must examine basic dimensions of language. Primary among these are use (pragmatics of the language), form (the grammatical or syntax aspect of language), and content (the semantic, vocabulary, or meaning aspect of the language). We suggest here that the childhood language disorder will very likely be found in one or a combination of these three dimensions of language. Review Figure 2.2, illustrating the capacities for normal language development, to recall the interrelationship of these dimensions.

Prevalence

How frequently this oral communication problem occurs in the population is not well known. In the distant past, language disorders were not considered part of the speech-language pathologist's domain. Now, language problems not only have become important targets for remediation, but have garnered large numbers of clinicians and researchers who specialize in this area. The national professional society that was earlier known as the American Speech and Hearing Association changed its name in 1978 to acknowledge the intensity of interest in this area: the American Speech-Language-Hearing Association. Language has become its middle name!

One early study estimating the number of children having language problems was done on a population of three-year-olds. Although the criteria for including a child in one category or another were rather broad, it appeared that about 30 children of each 1,000 had some form of language delay. Thus, about 3% might have been involved. Note that this study of three-year-old children used as its criteria rather broad language expectations. As uncertain as we are about the numbers, there is a real

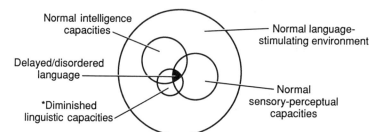

A The effect of diminshed linguistic capacities* on the development of language (compare with Fig. 2.2)

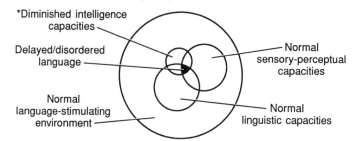

B The effect of diminished intelligence capacities* on the development of language

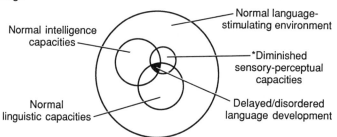

C The effect of diminshed sensory-perceptual capacities* on the development of language

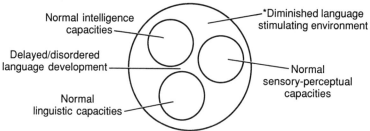

D The effect of diminished language-stimulating environment* on the development of speech

Figure 2.4.   Effects on Language Development of Diminished Capacities

consensus among professionals that children's language disorders are among the most common impairments in the development of a child.

> Practically speaking, what could the incidence figures mean? Using the 3% figure and applying it to a fairly large public school system having, say, 50,000 children, one might expect to find some 1,500 children with some form of language problem. In a smaller district of, say, 10,000 youngsters, there might be some 300 children that are delayed in language abilities. In an even smaller district of 5,000 children, only about 150 might be having such difficulties. The difference in numbers of children would point to differences in size of language programs and in the amount of budget allocation to such programs and to the hiring of specialists in language remediation. But, whether it is 150 or 1,500, the fact remains that these children are in need of help.

Some school districts have organized staff, rooms, facilities, and supporting personnel to assist in the remediation of language problems in older children. Teenagers having such problems can find themselves meeting a world of high expectations upon leaving the school setting. Schools are now attempting to provide tutorial and special remedial programs for such children. In some locales, these programs are identified as "language classes," the "aphasia program," the "specific language disorders center," and by other names.

Children's language disorders are the concern of Public Law 94–142 (the Education for All Handicapped Children Act of 1975). The terminology therein refers to "learning disabled children." Because *language* delay or disorder may be a large part of the *learning* disorder, attention may be placed upon the language aspect. Confusion arises, however, in what the problem is called. A variety of terms exist: developmental aphasia or dysphasia, specific language disability or disorder, language delay or disorder, delayed language development, and so on. Perhaps, as some authorities have suggested, a combined term should be adopted, such as language-learning disabled or disordered.

Characteristics

What are some of the "common characteristics" of children's language disorders? Because of the many dimensions to language learning—and disorders—there is considerable variation in these characteristics. Adding to this the fact that the severity of the disorder ranges from mild to severe, one might conclude that "characterizing" children's language disorders is a difficult task.

If we start by noting categories of characteristics, we find that the *modality* aspect varies, so that there are receptive, expressive, and processing language problems, and combinations of these. Examining the *dimensions* of language, one might find form, use, or content disorders. Considering *causality,* one might find children's language disorders stemming from (or associated with) such problems as mental retardation or hearing impairment; these are labeled *secondary* language disorders. In these, a primary problem produces several (secondary) disorders, among which may be language delay. On the other hand, we may find no causal basis for the language delay; it in itself is the *primary* language disorder. When the cause of the language disorder is unknown, it is called ideopathic.

There is a considerable range in the *severity* aspect of language disorders. Having a language disorder does not indicate a total absence of language, although this degree of severity may occur in a profoundly affected child. More often, however, children have only minimal language delays, perhaps measured in terms of a few months below expected age level performance. Standardized language assessment tests may show greater degrees of delay: moderate, moderately severe, or severe. The *effect* upon the child should be noted, from interpersonal relationships to academic skill and progress.

> Inasmuch as a five-year-old should have a fair grasp of language, it was quite apparent that Amelia showed a delay in language acquisition and use. As her kindergarten day ended, she was heard to say "Me go Momma." Analyzing this utterance, one sees errors in grammar and vocabulary, and a certain deficiency in what one might expect a child of that age to say in the social context. Although not a "fair" comparison, how would you frame a statement at the end of your working day?

In this last illustration, social content was mentioned. One might add to this the linguistic or communicative context. These are important constituents of pragmatics. When someone says "It's cold," the specific intent is not clear until one understands the context and the listener's background information at that moment. The intent could be (1) to speak about the weather outside, (2) to complain about the food, (3) to describe ice, (4) to request that the heat be turned on, or (5) to demand that the window be shut, among other things. What "It's cold" is used for thus depends upon who the speaker is, who the listener is, what both know, what the intention of the speaker is in affecting the listener, and the characteristics of the environment (context).

Language use requires certain abilities in the individual, among which are the ability to perceive the totality of a situation, or the context, and a fairly good grasp of the form of language and its meaning.

> There were times when William's parents were very confused about his utterances. "What did he mean?" was often expressed, even though he was quite articulate in forming most speech sounds. At times, when asked if he would like to go out to play, he might say something apparently unrelated, out of context, such as "Stars in rug are pretty." At other times, he might repeat what was said to him: "—like to go out to play—like to go out to play—like to go out to play," not meaning an affirmative response. His expressive *use* of language could have stemmed from confused language programming, as well as other conditions.

Thus a primary language disorder might be characterized as involving largely content, or form, or use, or some combination of these three aspects of language. The potential variability of problems among children is indeed considerable. The most common area in delayed language development is probably syntactic; many children demonstrate difficulty in acquiring skill in grammatical forms. Yet, content problems are also common, as for example in vocabulary paucity. When looking at a child with a language disorder it is clearly important to study the language problem itself. After all, to be of assistance to such a child requires knowledge of what is lacking.

> Jody, with a primary language disorder, is a healthy, vibrant little four-year-old, but her parents and friends find her extremely difficult to have around. Offering Jody something special, such as going for a ride or visiting Aunt Susie or going outside to play on the swing, often elicits a blank expression and no response. Then, taking the initiative, the adult suggests that Jody go to her room, select a sweater, and meet the adult at the front door. In response, Jody moves in the general direction of her room and then slows, stops, perhaps to be distracted by something else in the environment. The adult may then get the sweater and ask Jody to identify it. Minimal reactions from Jody may ensue: "sweater," "outside," "cold"; single-word responses may indicate that she is aware of the simplest meanings, but has some problem in associating the different components. Although otherwise intact, Jody has a truly primary language disorder.

As noted earlier, some types of language disorders are not primary but are secondary to another problem. One example of this is the language problem demonstrated by children said to be "mentally retarded." In the normal child, language age is usually commensurate with the mental age.

The term "mental retardation" refers to the functioning of a child under 18 years with less-than-average general intellectual performance and deficits or impairments in adaptive behavior. This below-average functioning is accompanied by below-peer levels of personal independence and social responsibilities. Intellectual functioning is usually determined by standardized intelligence tests, such as the Stanford Binet or the Wechsler, from which are derived IQ (intelligence quotient) scores. The test scores, the IQ that is developed from one of these examinations, are used to classify mental retardation. These tests differ somewhat in the actual IQ placement, but in general they follow the scheme shown in Table 2.5. Mental retardation is an uncommon and variable problem. Only about 2% of the entire population falls into this category; that is, some 98% of people have average or above-average intelligence.

The degree or severity of a child's language disorder is probably in proportion to the degree of mental retardation. One might expect a child with lowered cognitive

Table 2.5. Classification of Mental Retardation

IQ SCORE	CLASSIFICATION
62–84	Borderline
52–69 [a]	Mild
36–54 [a]	Moderate
20–39 [a]	Severe
Below 20	Profound

[a] There is an overlap in ranges here because the higher IQ score is from one test and the lower from the other (see text).

abilities to begin to use and develop skill in language at a later age than an otherwise average child. Vocabulary, syntactic skill, and complexity increases are slower than in children of a comparable chronologic age. Children who are mentally retarded often have limited linguistic abilities and more simplified language use. It is often difficult to accelerate language skills to chronologic age levels. Language skills might be improved to approximate mental age, but not chronologic age.

Figure 2.5 is a graphic illustration of delay in certain developmental areas compared with chronologic age. Thus language age, as measured by standardized tests, might well be less than chronologic age: this is delayed language development. Mental age, as measured by standardized intelligence testing, may also be less than chronologic age. Phoneme mastering, another skill to be developed in oral communication, will be considered in detail in Chapter 3, but is introduced at this point to illustrate the many other developmental abilities that a child must master.

> Fred was born with a significant degree of mental retardation. At the outset, it was evident that Fred was not developing as rapidly as other children of his age group. Some of his motor skills, including walking and feeding himself, were slow in developing and remained uncoordinated and clumsy. When other children were saying their first words, somewhere around their first birthdays, Fred was not. As other children, around kindergarten age, were completing sentences, using plurals and possessives, Fred was still using one-word utterances with only occasional two-word expressions. Fred was developing language according to his mental age, not his chronologic age. The language disorder was secondary to his intellectual retardation.

Another secondary language disorder is that which follows *hearing loss* in the important language-acquisition years. Both speech and language are learned largely

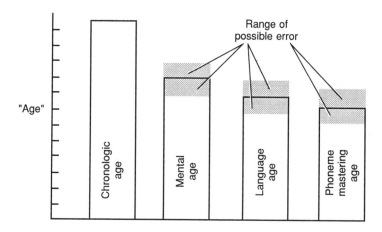

Figure 2.5.   Reduced Mental, Language, and Phoneme Mastering* Ages Compared with Chronologic Age
* Phoneme mastering is discussed in Chapter 3.

through auditory avenues. Whatever speech and language children actually hear from their "talking" environment form the model for their own developing speech and language. Each child makes his/her own communication attempts on the model in his/her mind. The child who is born with absolutely no hearing would develop no oral language through the usual language learning means. In general, with less of a hearing problem, or with one occurring later in the language learning period, there would be less of a language disorder. The language disorder is secondary to and commensurate with the degree of auditory disorder. The types, degrees, and effects of auditory disorders will be discussed more extensively in later chapters.

> Jenny had a serious infectious disease shortly after her birth. She incurred a long period of elevated temperatures; she was treated with several pharmaceutical agents to preserve her life, but lost her hearing in the process. It slowly became apparent after her illness that she was not responding to sound in her environment. She did not startle at loud sounds; she did not respond to the different voices of her parents; she did not seem to seek the source of unusual sounds such as rattles and bells in her crib area. She also did not respond to what people said to her. As she grew older, it became evident that she did not understand what was said to her, although her other abilities seemed adequate for her age level. She could walk and run and do puzzles and draw pictures and engage in many other activities of "normal" children. But she did not follow oral instructions and she did not start using words. Her vocal efforts were more like grunts or squeals or other unspeechlike sounds than words. With her severe hearing loss she could not perceive the language stimuli around her. Since a model for developing her own oral speech and language did not exist, such development did not occur. Jenny's deafness was primary to her secondary language disorder.

Another source of language problems is that associated with a child's *emotional state.* True psychologic or personality disorders such as childhood psychosis may indeed be accompanied by language disorders. In some instances, the child's personality disorder is first noted as a problem in oral communication. Although considerable variability exists in the language disorders exhibited by children with personality aberrations, one outstanding kind of problem is in the use area of language. The language may prove to be quite inappropriate to the situation of the moment. For example, it has been said that these children "talk" but do not "communicate." Such children might also demonstrate a content problem, showing some errors in the meanings of words and expressions. It appears that they do not know what the words mean, for they select them in unusual ways. This semantic problem may be viewed as part of the pragmatic problem, until some careful and thorough testing is done to isolate the two aspects of oral communication.

Autism is a problem closely allied to communication skills. Some authorities insist that this disorder cannot be diagnosed unless language is analyzed. Certainly, an autistic youngster may not establish a meaningful communicative exchange. Whether autism is a true psychosis or is related to aphasia or some other behavioral problem stemming from another etiologic condition is not a matter of great agreement. The unusual speech and language characteristics often observed in this condition include parrotlike, even *echolalic* (meaningless repetitions), made-up words, pronoun confusions, and unusual prosodic (melody and stress) patterns in speech.

> Whatever the cause, Ronnie's language was said to be bizarre. Often people heard his words as intelligible, but the meaning of what he was saying sometimes just failed to come through. When asked if he wanted a cookie or an apple, Ronnie might seem to respond with "Turn on the light." Or, he could as easily fail to respond orally, but simply turn and walk away, or hide his eyes, or otherwise avoid the speaker. If, when Ronnie was busily engaged in playing with a toy, someone asked what he was doing, again he might avoid answering completely or seem to respond to the query with an out-of-context statement. It would not be unusual for Ronnie to make up a word, a jargon term, that would be meaningless to his listener. His self-talking times (as when he talked with his toys when alone) could easily relate to an entirely different situation from whatever he might be doing at that moment.

Emotional problems in adults can result in parallel effects on language. In the case of the child, interference with use of language can also affect many learning activities through which a child must pass. Unusual personal and social behaviors may be observed. Associated with language delay and behavioral differences may be other delays, for example in reading.

One might look to other possible causal factors associated with children's language disorders, some intrinsic to the child, some extrinsic. The health and stability of the nervous system, for example, may be another broadly related area. One may find different degrees, types, and durations of brain injuries and damaging neurologic influences in the histories of some language-delayed children. Other intrinsic negative influences also occur, for example in the chronically ill child or the one with severe physical trauma, such as in burn or accident cases. A secondary language delay might be identified in a youngster with important decrements in the social-affective environment—an extrinsic cause. Although perhaps otherwise intrinsically normal and capable of learning language, a child in a non-language-stimulating environment, for example, may well be delayed in this learned behavior. The "talking" environment triggers language behavior. Failure to be in such a social-affective environment is thus importantly related to slow language development.

EVALUATION

Before any problem is "treated" or managed, one should not only determine the nature of the problem in its various aspects, but also identify the causes, if such can be found. This is no less true for human communication disorders. Because children's language delays or disorders offer so many dimensions, a careful evaluation may be complex.

It is important for the speech-language pathologist to determine the language dimensions involved. Does the child have problems primarily in the content area? Or in the form of his/her language? In the area of use, does the youngster grasp inferences and generalities and utilize pragmatics as another child of the same age might?

Knowing which dimension may be disturbed certainly initiates the management direction: what should be enhanced?

The speech-language pathologist should explore the various aspects of language and language development in order to get some sort of baseline information on language understanding, processing, and expression. Standardized procedures are the safest to use in all aspects, if at all possible. For example, the standard way of determining the mean length of utterance was described earlier, and that approach should be followed each time.

The specialist utilizes other approaches in evaluating the child, his/her language abilities, and the environment in which the child lives. Not only are language samples taken—the clinician observing the child in a communicative setting (e.g., the child and his/her mother playing and talking in a clinical room)—but an interview with the parent(s) offers considerable additional information. A history of the child's development, especially linguistic development but including other developmental landmarks (e.g., walking, toilet training), can offer a good deal of helpful information. Health history, family changes, and variations in living situation are some of the influences on child language development.

In some clinics, language diaries are used. As part of the total evaluation, the child's daily language performances can be noted by a parent or other adult. Check sheets and even tape-recorded samples may be made for later evaluation by the speech-language pathologist.

All of these approaches, and much more, add clinical data that increase one's knowledge about the child and his/her language problem. From that knowledge will come a better informed management (or treatment) program.

GENERAL MANAGEMENT APPROACHES

The older term for guiding or assisting a person to better communication skills is "therapy" or "treatment"; more and more the preferred term is becoming "management." It is directed activity, not just hands-on activity taking place in a clinic room. Clinic room "therapy" does occur, of course. Sometimes it takes place as a demonstration for an observing parent or teacher. Directions may then be given for the activities to be reinforced at home or in a playroom or classroom; diaries of what occurs may be requested. The pathologist can then assess the efficacy of the management program by examining written and oral reports as well as by evaluating changes in the child's linguistic behavior in a clinic room. Management does not have to be restricted to a clinic environment. It can occur in any environment that might prove to be stimulating and rewarding to the youngster's talking efforts.

A child whose language is delayed in development should receive guidance in such ways that he/she can use language effectively in everyday life. Goals are established that accommodate several aspects involved in the disorder. One is to consider those dimensions of language that are below average; if the problem is syntax, then grammatical forms are taught and encouraged, for example. Another aspect to consider is causality; intervention for a child with a primary language delay would differ somewhat from that for a child with a severe hearing impairment that is primary to the language delay.

So, not only are goals laid out, but the means of achieving these goals must be planned. Goals are both long- and short-term in expectation. Long-term goals include the larger one: the effective use of language in everyday life. Short-term goals are steps along the way; for example, teaching and stimulating the use of possessives ("Daddy's hat"). As the management program continues, objective and quantitative assessment of progress must be made. From such assessment come adjustments and changes in procedures, whether they occur in the "therapy room" or are encouraged in a classroom or in the home by other members of the management team: the classroom teacher or aide, the parent, or other family member.

SUMMARY

Children's language disorders are often characterized as a delay in the development of language skills. The delay is often scaled upon the child's chronologic age. If one of the prerequisite capacities for language acquisition is less than adequate, one might expect a commensurate less-than-adequate language development skill. These are secondary delays. A "delay" suggests that the child is slower in moving through a developmental language sequence.

A language disorder, on the other hand, indicates a gap in the child's language acquisition. Some aspects may be adequate, but in another there is a significant lacking. A child with a basic emotional problem or with an important neurologic (brain) disorder or dysfunction could well demonstrate a language disorder.

Language structure falls into three linguistic dimensions: meaning (semantics), form (syntax), and use (pragmatics). Problems in one or more of these areas can point to certain bases or underlying problems in other characteristics of the youngster. The speech-language pathologist determines whether the child's language problem is in the area of meaning, structure, or use. One can then determine what might be behind the problem.

Etiologic studies of children center around the analysis of the prerequisite capacities for linguistic development. The levels of intellectual, sensory-perceptual, and inborn linguistic capacities are determined. One or more of these might well underlie the language problem. Further, it is essential to understand the stimulating environment for the child. Knowing this allows one to establish prognostic estimates and even to select remediation approaches appropriate not only to the problem but to the capacities of the child. Such approaches are often highly individualistic, with only some similarities among approaches for large numbers of children.

Language disorders in children are not always primary problems and are not always the only problem the child has. The language problems of some children are secondary to other, more basic, problems. Outstanding among them are auditory disorders, mental retardation, and emotional difficulties. It is important to identify whether the language problem is primary or secondary when considering remediation. The problem must be analyzed in terms of its language dimensions so that one can set goals and targets for remediation.

Considerable study in all aspects of children's language disorders has already taken place and will certainly continue. It is important that such disorders be identified as early as possible to prevent the development of secondary and tertiary side effects. Problems may occur in the educational, social, vocational, and other aspects of the individual's life as he/she grows and develops in a society that demands verbal skills for success.

SUGGESTED READINGS

Brown, R. (1973). *A First Language: The Early Stages.* Cambridge, MA: Harvard University Press. *Roger Brown's work in child language development established a pattern of quantitatively documenting stages and of qualitatively describing those stages. This text is but one of a multitude of writings that have stimulated research and clinical management resulting in a considerable body of experience and knowledge.*

Chomsky, N. (1972). *Language and Mind.* New York: Harcourt Brace Jovanovich. *The name of Chomsky evokes both respect and questioning attitudes, but certainly this and his other writings have done much to stimulate research and hypotheses in the field of human language use.*

Dale, P. (1976). *Language Development: Structure and Function,* 2nd ed. New York: Holt, Rinehart & Winston. *A major and authoritative presentation of the subject from an important researcher in the field. The text is comprehensive, factual, and thorough in its coverage.*

Lahey, M. (1988). *Language Disorders and Language Development.* New York: Macmillan. *The revised book Language Development and Language Disorders by Lois Bloom and Margaret Lahey. Both texts will serve the beginning student, expanding considerably upon basic information. As Lahey states, her text "presumes that students have had some introductory course work in language development." It remains a helpful and authoritative book.*

Miller, J.F. (1981). *Assessing Language Production in Children.* Baltimore: University Park Press. *An objective and quantitative approach to the study of the language skills of children.*

Reed, V.A. (1986). *An Introduction to Children with Language Disorders.* New York: Macmillan. *An interesting beginning survey of children and their language, delay, and broadly related aspects.*

Study Questions

1. Search for a definition of perception, not in a dictionary, and use that definition in describing how a child learns to use the language that people speak all around him/her. You might have to ignore some of the personal capacities required as you focus upon perceptual skills.

2. Describe the status of an adult who was delayed in language development as a child. What kinds of work might such a person have? What hobbies or avocations or interests? What subjects would you guess might have been difficult, and which easy, when this person was in high school? Did he/she graduate?

3. If a child shows important language delay because of profound hearing impairment, how might a teacher or other person communicate language concepts? If you think some form of sign language might be helpful, what do you know about its own linguistic structure? Is there a syntax?

4. A blue jay shrieks in response to the presence of an intruder; a chimpanzee chatters about the arrival of food; a dog growls when another of its kind approaches. How would you label actions of this type? Do they constitute language? Is communication occurring? Does communication have to be linguistic?

5. If language use is an activity centered somewhere in the brain, what do you think of the possibility that an adult might suffer a brain injury and lose language skill? Does it happen? (See Chapter 5, "Neurogenic Disorders.") If it does happen, could it take place in one of the linguistic dimensions: semantic, syntax, or pragmatics? Or would it be a fairly widespread sort of loss?

6. How do you think a speech-language pathologist might objectively (even quantitatively) evaluate the progress that a child with delayed language might make as a result of teaching or therapy? Would it be best to develop some new form as a "yardstick," or should one use the same tests used in the initial evaluation of the child's language use?

3

Articulation/Phonology Disorders

A type of communication disorder that is fairly common among persons of all ages is associated with the act of articulated speech. Normal articulation means the production of acceptable speech-sounds of various types as most people use them. These sounds, the phonetic aspect of speech, are classified by phoneticians as to their individual characteristics and how they may be combined in actual speech, as dictated by governing phonologic rules. These two dimensions, the nature of the speech sounds themselves and the linguistic rules regulating the use of the speech sounds, suggest two different types of speech-sound errors: phonetic and phonologic. Phonemes are learned by children over a fair number of years, even into the second grade. Delays in phoneme learning, exemplified in several ways, result in articulation disorders. A person of any age can display such a disorder. Differing causes underlie different problems. Assessment explores the types, severity, and causes of articulation disorders, and provides directions toward management methods. Phonologic errors refer to speech-sound disorders associated with how the sounds are used, closely allied to the linguistic rules that might be broken. In this chapter, we mainly consider phonetic or articulation errors, but phonologic errors are also important.

INTRODUCTION

As described in Chapter 2, *language* is the "code" in human communication, the symbolic formulation of messages to be uttered (or written, or signed). In uttering the message, the sender uses standard (in his/her own language group such as English or Russian) elements, *phonemes* or *speech-sounds*. In general, these are the vowels and consonants of a language. The process of producing those sounds, resulting in meaningful language morphemes, words, phrases, etc., is *articulation*. The specific language (e.g., English or Russian) utilizes a limited number of accepted speech sounds. Each language has its own rules about the use of its phonemes. These are the *phonologic* aspects, the linguistic rules and customs of phoneme use (*phonology*).

Articulation disorders are thought to be the most common of all the communication disorders. They are errors in the way that people say the speech-sounds of their language. Because there seems to be a generally accepted, normal way of articulation, anything other than this is considered a disorder.

Accurate estimates of prevalence are difficult to find. Most figures stem from surveys performed in public schools and in controlled populations such as college freshmen who are screened as part of their entrance procedures. In 1981, ASHA (the journal of the American Speech-Language-Hearing Association) reported the overall prevalence of articulation errors in public school children as 1.9%. In itself, this may seem a surprisingly small figure, but it came from a survey of over 38,000 school children in grades 1 through 12. As you might expect, there are different prevalences at each grade level. In this study, almost 10% of first grade children demonstrated articulation errors. The figure dropped by half to about 5% at grade 2, dropped again by more than half to 2.0% by grade 3, and subsequently decreased in smaller steps until only 0.5% of the group in grade 12 were found to have articulation errors.

Some children seem to be slower in learning normal articulatory skills, but most do seem to master this speech necessity. By grade 12, as children enter adulthood, a few retain articulation or phonologic problems. Although careful screening of all adults has not been done, it appears from these figures (as well as from the experience of many speech clinicians) that articulation errors may be found in persons of all ages.

THE SYMBOL SYSTEM: PHONETICS

Introduction

The speech-sounds of our language parallel in part the letters of our alphabet. In fact, the alphabet was developed so that we could write what we say. What we say consists of *vowels* and *consonants* embedded in a framework of *prosody: pitch, rate, melody,* and *loudness* of voice. In general, speech-sounds (or *phonemes*) are uttered in groups called words, then phrases, and then sentences, and so on. The phoneme is not a limited unit, such as a meter or a pound, but is a small group or family of sounds (or phones) that can be identified in a rather singular, symbolic way. For example, not all the /s/-type sounds (a hissing sound, not the name of the alphabet letter) are identical, nor are all the /a/ or /t/ sounds. (Note that phoneme symbols are placed in slash marks.) The /s/ phoneme or speech-sound is heard in words such as "sister," "pass," "stew," "seem," and "pest" in which the alphabet letter *s* does represent the sound. The alphabet letter *s* is spoken as a different sound, however, in the words "pays," or "rose," or "pigs"; in these cases, the speech-sound is /z/, a fraternal twin to /s/ perhaps. Also, the /s/ phoneme is often "spelled" with a *c,* as in "cinnamon." Even so, not all /s/ phonemes are articulated (spoken) exactly the same way, for they may differ slightly according to their place in syllables or may even be articulated slightly differently by different people. With groups of friends, we identify families by family names such as the "Rodriguez" or the "Abercrombies." We know that each member of the family is not identical to each other member; calling them "Abercrombie" is simply a manner of saying they belong to each other in several unique ways. The same sort of thing applies to speech-sounds. The phoneme is a closely related family of speech-sounds, such as /s/, that may not be identical to each other, but are "close enough" to carry the same phonetic symbol.

Phonemes are very nearly alike throughout a language. They are studied in courses on phonetics. We can talk about phonemes and we can write about them, using a symbol system that represents the spoken phoneme. Phoneticians and others use the International Phonetic Alphabet. In each language, only a part of the total international number of symbols may be used, so in English there is a shortened version of the larger alphabet as described by Tiffany and Carrell (see Suggested Readings). The phonemes of our language (Table 3.1) are commonly of two kinds: vowels and consonants. The larger acoustic differences between the two types of speech-sounds stem from the way the chambers and structures of the neck and head are utilized to modify the raw sounds of voice and flowing air (Fig. 3.1).

Table 3.1. The American English Phonetic Alphabet

PHONETIC SYMBOL	WORD EXAMPLE	PHONETIC SYMBOL	WORD EXAMPLE	PHONETIC SYMBOL	WORD EXAMPLE
CONSONANTS					
Those with Phonetic Symbols the Same as Alphabet Symbols					
/p/	pan	/f/	fan	/m/*	map
/b/*	ban	/v/*	van	/n/*	nap
/t/	tan	/s/	sip	/l/*	lap
/d/*	Dan	/z/*	zip	/w/*	wag
/k/	kit	/h/	hip	/r/*	rip
/g/*	gag				
Those with Phonetic Symbols Different from Alphabet Symbols					
/θ/	ether	/ʒ/*	azure	/ŋ/*	Chang
/ð/*	either	/tʃ/	church	/hw/	when
/ʃ/	shin	/dʒ/*	George		
VOWELS					
Front		Central		Back	
High /i/	east	/ɝ/	bird	/u/	suit
/ɪ/	sit	/ɚ/	other	/U/	soot
/e/	state	/ʌ/	cup	/O/	coat
/ɛ/	said	/ə/	alone	/ɒ/	cot
Low /æ/	sat			/ɔ/	caught

* Voiced consonants.

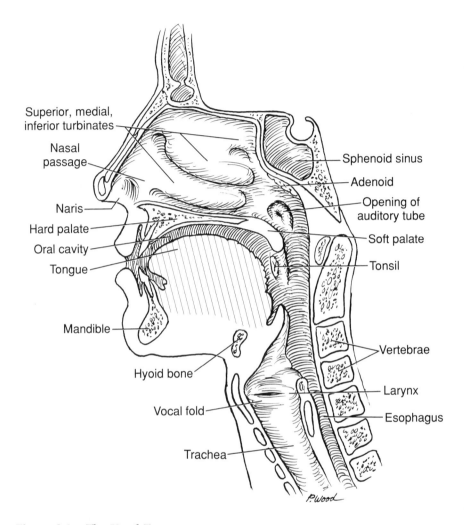

Superior, medial, inferior turbinates
Nasal passage
Naris
Hard palate
Oral cavity
Tongue
Mandible
Hyoid bone
Vocal fold
Trachea

Sphenoid sinus
Adenoid
Opening of auditory tube
Soft palate
Tonsil
Vertebrae
Larynx
Esophagus

P. Wood

Figure 3.1. The Vocal Tract.
From Palmer, J. M. (1984). *Anatomy for Speech and Hearing,* 3rd ed. New York: Harper & Row.

Articulation of Vowels and Consonants

Vowels are modifications of the vocal tone after it is produced at the vocal folds. Vowels are *resonance phenomena.* This suggests that the vocal folds have produced the raw material, a vocal tone. This tone is then modified or resonated acoustically into the different vowels by the series of chambers above the vocal folds. Resonance changes occur because the lower jaw (mandible bone) moves up or down to change the relative mouth position of the tongue, up or down. The tongue can then effect smaller changes in the mouth chamber (oral cavity proper), in the volume as well as the contour (shape) of the cavity. Such changes are heard as vowels. They occur because anatomic structures, the several articulators, move to change the dimensions of the mouth and throat resulting in different resonated sounds (Fig. 3.1).

Vowels are classified by the posture of the tongue. The tongue postures become vowel *features*. Individual vowel sounds are identified as "high front," or "mid vowels," or "low back," etc., depending upon what the tongue does within the oral cavity (see Fig. 7.2) to change the resonance chamber, for vowels are resonance phenomena. (A further description of resonance is included in the discussion of voice and voice production in Chapter 4.) If the tongue is lifted high and relatively toward the front of the mouth, the resulting vowel is called a *high front vowel.* Table 3.2 shows which vowels are the highest and the most front. The appropriate phonetic symbol as well as a single-syllable word using that vowel are also included. Keeping the tongue high, but this time more toward the back of the mouth, causes the vowel to be a *high back vowel.* Examine the vowel diagram and the illustrative words (Table 3.2) and identify, in general, the tongue movements used as you make those sounds, those vowels.

We can also cause the blending of two (or even more) vowels into *diphthongs.* Subtle changes of the tongue during vowel production cause a shift in the nature of the speech-sound. For example, the word "out" commences with a vowel similar to *ah* but moves smoothly to a vowel nearly *oo,* or using the International Phonetic Alphabet, from /a/ to /u/ in a single dynamic action. The word is then terminated with the consonant spelled with the English alphabet letter *t,* and phonetically /t/, similar in orthography but different in referent. The diphthong here is /au/, although some speakers use /ɔ ʊ/ in such instances; variation among normal speakers is common.

Table 3.2. Physiologic Vowel Diagram

	Front	Central	Back
High	i (heed)	(you)* iu/ju	u (hoot)
	I (hid)		U (hood)
Mid	e (hate)		o (hoe)
		ʌ (hut) / ə (sofa)	ɔɪ (boy)*
		ɝ (bird) / ɚ (other)	
	ɛ (head)	au (house)	ɑ (father)
Low	æ (had)		ɔ (hod)

ai (high)

Ms. Popovich (or Ms. Partucci, or Ms. Simone) studied English in her native country and was nearly perfect in grammar, syntax, and pragmatics. However, it was not difficult for a native American speaker to recognize that she was not a native American speaker, and to even guess her Slavic (or Italian, or French) background. For example, the uncommon /I/ sound in American English is often uttered (by non-American speakers) as /i/. Thus, words such as "mit," or "hit," or "bit," for example, would be heard as "meet," or "heat," or "beet." In practice, the non-American speaker heard, and uttered, the /i/ sound in all cases, for that was a common vowel in her native language; /I/ may not have occurred at all.

Consonant articulation often requires a tonal quality (voicing) as well as the flow and pressure of exhaled air through the mouth. There are two types of sound we can use in one of three different manners: (1) voicing; (2) not voicing, but using the sound of air as we control it; and (3) combining the two to produce a voiced airstream sound. Voicing (or its absence) is one of three *features* of consonant production. A feature is a required aspect.

We continue to rely heavily on the mandible and the tongue as primary *articulators*. Other articulators besides the tongue are the lips, the teeth, the ridge in which the teeth reside (alveolar ridge), the hard palate immediately behind that ridge, and the movable soft palate (velum) at the back of the mouth. Consonant articulation requires a relatively constricted (sometimes closed) vocal tract, bringing one articulator close to another to modify airstream as well as vocal tone, when present. Modification produces different types of consonants.

The three features of consonant sounds can now be identified: where anatomically the constriction takes place (*placement*), what kind (*manner*) of sound results, and whether or not *voicing* occurs in phone production. In Table 3.3 these three features are used as a classification system. For example, if the placement of a sound is described as linguadental, it means that the tongue (*lingua-*) approaches the teeth (*dental*) in placement. Note the other terms describing the *placement* of phonemes in Table 3.3. Bilabial refers to two (*bi-*) lips (*labial*); labiodental, lip (*labio-*) to teeth (*dental*); lingua-alveolar, tongue (*lingua-*) to the alveolar ridge; linguapalatal, tongue (*lingua-*) to the hard palate; linguavelar, tongue (*lingua-*) toward the soft palate (*velar*) to change the vocal system in producing whatever consonant is referred to. (See Fig. 3.1 to locate anatomic landmarks.)

To identify the *manner* of sound, we use speech-sound classification terms (Table 3.3). These terms refer to the types of acoustic events produced as we move the articulators from place to place, while exhaling and perhaps *voicing*. Thus, there is a *stop* sound, meaning that the consonant is the result of the system being arrested or stopped. Note in Table 3.3 that the /p/ sound, as well as the /t/ and /k/, are *stops*. These three phonemes, /p/, /t/, and /k/, do not utilize voice as we make them. They are termed "*voiceless*" or "unvoiced" speech-sounds. Should we add that voicing feature, we would produce the voiced counterparts of those three sounds: /b/, /d/, and /g/.

Another type of speech-sound is the *fricative*. Perhaps to the reader this term implies "friction," and it is indeed a friction product. The exhaled airstream through the oral cavity proper can be directed toward articulators (teeth, alveolar ridge,

Table 3.3. Consonant Production

PLACE OF ARTICULATION	MANNER OF ARTICULATION				
	STOP	FRICATIVE	AFFRICATE	LATERAL/ GLIDE	NASAL
Bilabial	p, b*			hw, w*	m*
Labiodental		f, v*			
Linguadental		θ, ð*			
Lingua-alveolar	t, d*	s, z*		l*	n*
Linguapalatal		ʃ, ʒ*	tʃ, dʒ*	j*, r*	
Linguavelar	k, g*				ŋ*
Glottal		h			

Adapted from Fisher, H. and J. Logemann (1971). *The Fisher-Logemann Test of Articulation Competence*. Boston: Houghton Mifflin.
* Voiced consonants.

palate) by the tongue. The flowing, pressurized air forced through some constriction at some locale becomes turbulent and noisy. This sound is identified as a consonant. For example, lifting the tongue tip toward the alveolar ridge or the teeth and causing a somewhat narrow stream of air to strike one or the other results in a hissing or sibilant sound: the /s/ phoneme. Moving the tongue more posteriorly and flattening its upper surface (dorsum) causes the turbulent sound to be "broader." This is the sound one utters when hushing another person, in English *sh,* but in the phonetic symbol system, /ʃ/. Another fricative, /f/, is produced by elevating the lower lip to the edge of the upper teeth while flowing pressurized air passes through the constricted area. Examples of each of these, in order, are "seat," "sheet," and "feet." Each has its voiced cognate, of course, as in "zoo," "measure," and "oven."

Yet another sound is the *th* speech-sound. Its phonetic symbol is /θ/. In the word "thin," the first sound is unvoiced but is produced by introducing the tongue tip slightly between the upper and lower teeth, allowing a gentle flow of air to pass the constriction there. The turbulence in the air, a friction sound, establishes the characteristic fricative. There is a voiced cognate, as in the word "either."

One last fricative sound is the *glottal* /h/. The adjective "glottal" refers to the airway between the two vocal folds (glottis). This sound is made when the vocal folds come somewhat near each other so that air is forced between the constriction in a turbulent fashion. The resulting fricative is the product of the articulatory placement of the folds within the airstream. The airstream during exhalation for nonspeech breathing otherwise is not an audible sound. One might note, too, that the vocal folds are utilized in this sound production but are not always called articulators. This sound, /h/, is often classified as a glide rather than a fricative.

Another consonant sound type is the *affricate.* This sound has a friction component combined with a stop characteristic: thus, the /tʃ/ (as in "watch"), and its voiced counterpart /dʒ/ (as in "judge").

Yet another group of sounds are the *laterals* or *glides.* The lateral /l/ and the /r/

are often classified in this group. The glides are /w/, /j/, and /h/ and sometimes /hw/. The term "liquid" is sometimes used for lateral. Review Table 3.1 for the complete list and representative words for each consonant and vowel.

Another of the phoneme group is the *nasal* trio. "Nasal" indicates that the speech-producing system is sending voicing into the nasal passages (as well as the mouth) to effect the unique nature of the sounds. The /m/ and /n/ sounds are nasal consonants. The first is made by placing together the upper and lower lips while voicing a nasally resonated sound. The second is produced by elevating the tongue tip to the alveolar ridge, or thereabouts, and again allowing the sound being produced to enter the nasal region. The third member of the trio is the /ŋ/ sound. This is commonly identified, by nonphoneticians of course, as the *ng* sound. It is always embedded within a word or terminates (or arrests) the word, as in "hanger" or "sing." In these cases, velopharyngeal closure does not occur; nasal chambers are coupled to oral chambers to create these nasal consonants.

Thus, the many different consonant phonemes are the product of a somewhat constricted vocal tract modifying either or both the flowing airstream and the vocal tone. The constriction is created by mobile articulators (e.g., lips, lower teeth, alveolar ridge, palate), while velopharyngeal closure directs air and vocal tone into the oral cavity (except in the case of the nasals).

> Mr. Phon was injured in an auto accident; part of his injuries involved tongue damage. He could not lift his tongue-tip, especially in fast-moving speech. As a result, Mr. Phon had difficulty producing /s/ and /z/ as well as other tongue-tip sounds. Because these were not present in his conversational speech, some listeners had difficulty understanding his spoken intentions, for the /s/ and /z/ are extremely common consonants in English.

PROSODY

Vowels and consonants are important segments of a spoken language. However, there is another component beyond the segment level (*suprasegmental*) that adds to the meaningfulness of an utterance. This component is also known as *prosody*. It occurs at both the word level and the sentence level. Authorities are not entirely agreed on the constituents of prosody, and terminology varies. In general, it refers to the melody or intonation of speech, the rhythm of the syllables or words, the loudness variations, the quality of the voice, and the duration of syllables. Much that is meaningful can be added to an utterance through prosody. The intentions of a speaker, the underlining of words or phrases, the emotionality of a spoken thought, and the forcefulness of a sentence are imparted through prosodic means. In contradistinction might be the utterances of machine-speech, a speaking robot, that has no built-in prosodic program.

DEVELOPMENT OF ARTICULATORY SKILLS

We now examine the developing child, especially how he/she begins to use the speech-sounds of the language. How do average or so-called normal children acquire sound after sound as they grow? First, we will look at those capacities necessary to acquire articulatory skill. When a child does not have articulatory skill, the speech-language pathologist attempts to identify which of these capacities might be behind the difficulty and then begins remediation using this as the guide.

Capacities Necessary for Articulatory Development

A considerable number of attributes can be listed to illustrate that the child developing speech skills must have a fairly sophisticated, well-organized, and adequate system. First, the child needs to have and use adequate intelligence, *cognitive adequacy.* Second, he/she must have *sensory adequacy,* with emphasis upon hearing abilities but also including the senses of touch, kinesthesis (movement), and proprioception (location of body parts). Third, *anatomic adequacy* is essential; the articulators listed earlier must be present to produce the speech sounds. Fourth, the functioning of the various parts with each other due to *neuromotor adequacy* is indeed important. Lastly, *environmental adequacy* is essential in that the developing child needs to live in a "talking" environment so that adequate models are available from which the youngster can pattern his/her own speech.

> The children seen by Mrs. Martin in her work as a speech pathologist included Jeanne, Inge, Johnny, Adam, and Pete. All had articulation problems, each different from the others and for different etiologic reasons. Jeanne, who was mentally retarded, used only two vowels and stop consonants. Inge, who had a long-standing hearing impairment, omitted nearly all fricatives and especially sibilants. Johnny's unrepaired cleft palate prevented him from controlling oral air flow and air pressure, so he produced almost no "pressure" consonants, especially stops. Adam, who had a form of cerebral palsy, was unable to effect the very fine muscle control for consonant production in normal rate of speech, and many words were unintelligible. Pete had been isolated from all other people as a child because of certain emotional problems in his mother, and he had nearly no speech stimulation as an infant; thus, his articulatory, as well as linguistic, vocabulary was extremely limited.

One might add to this list, of course. Perhaps these five capacities cover the necessary skill or attribute level for a child to learn to use the phonemes of his/her language. Among other characteristics one might consider is the child's personality or emotional status as it operates in a family or other circle of influence. Another possible characteristic is general body health, for example fatigue or enthusiasm levels and fluctuating health problems that may possibly influence speech development. However, assuming that the child has most of the prerequisite capacities for learning speech, one could expect the rate of acquiring phonetic skill to be within normal limits. At what ages, in general, can the child be expected to move through the speech-sound acquisition levels?

Chronologic Speech Development Patterns

All people do not develop in the same ways. Many aspects of growth and behavior vary considerably. Newborn infants have different birth weights, heights or lengths, and social environments. Differences continue throughout life. People grow taller at different rates. They develop skills at different ages. As speech skill development is discussed, it is important to remember that absolute ages (e.g., 13 months or five years) for developmental events cannot be specified. Instead, we discuss development in terms of *ranges* of ages. Individual differences can better be accommodated, and accepted, once this is understood.

Articulation (speech-sound production) skills commence early, postnatally, with the infant making perceptual judgments concerning the speech sounds of people in his/her environment. The young infant learns to pick out mother's voice from the dog's barking or the door closing or the kitchen food mixer running. This kind of sound discrimination is critical and is refined to finer and finer acts of auditory perception and discrimination. At a very early age, a few weeks in fact, the child can differentiate among some of the vowel and consonant sounds of the language. Ultimately, word discrimination creeps in. These perceptual skills precede the actual speaking acts that follow. The youngster's speech-sound production is an attempt to copy what he/she perceives.

Speech-sound production is preceded by much vocal activity, starting at the birth cry. Early infancy sounds such as cries, grunts, even screeches are products of the developing speech-language system. Refinements come along, especially when the child finds some reaction to the sounds he/she produces.

Early, the child utters many of the speech sounds in his/her environment. Sometimes this is entirely in babbling, in vocal play, in random utterances. Sometimes it may be more deliberate. We may well hear some very real speech sounds early in life; however, they may prove to be inconsistently used, appearing on some occasions and not on others. True acquisition of the use of a phoneme occurs when the child uses it correctly and regularly in words that require it.

To determine that a child is "at age level" in developing articulatory skill some normative data must have been collected: what does the normal or average child do in this respect? Over the years, a number of researchers have studied children to get such norms. Here, some generalizations and perhaps approximations will be given. Please recognize that there are different ways in which such studies can be made, and thus differences reported in how children learn to use the speech-sounds of their language.

Vowel acquisition comes fairly early in the development of phones. Although this has not been intensively studied, most clinicians accept the very early age of two years to 30 months, certainly no later than three years of age, as the age level by which the average child should have acquired mastery of all the vowels of his/her language. Consonant sound acquisition is another matter. Not only is there more variability in the norms, but it takes several more years for all consonant sounds to be mastered. At the outset, it should be clear that the average child will have been practicing and using many consonant sounds from the very beginnings of life. Cooing and babbling are some combination of vowels and consonants. As time moves on the youngster commonly uses some consonants correctly about 50% of the time. The 50% level is often used as a measuring stick. We say the sound is *customarily produced* at this level. The sounds *emerging* are becoming more usual than not.

From the beginning, Carla was quite normal in all aspects of development. This was especially true in speech development. Early on, before her first birthday, she "jabbered" happily to her toys, her food, her parents. If one analyzed Carla's speech throughout this period, one would hear all sorts of vowels and consonants in all sorts of combinations. For example, the /d/ phoneme appeared occasionally as in "duh," or "ada," etc. Once in a while, her parents heard what they considered to be a real word; Carla's father was especially delighted to hear her say "Dadda." Yet, she omitted the /d/ for "dog." But as she developed, she did start to use /d/ commonly, with frequent omissions still occurring. Carla *customarily* used /d/ when she was about two years of age, but it was not until she was four-years-old that she used it nearly all the time (90%), when she could be said to have *mastered* the sound.

A more realistic articulation skill level is when the child is said to have *mastered* the use of a particular phoneme. This is usually considered to be about the 90% level: 90% of the time that the child attempts to use a certain consonant, it is used correctly. There are norms for this level as well. Obviously this is the more useful score when comparing the child's articulation skills with those of the adult, but the 50% level is very helpful in considering the developing child who cannot be compared with the adult norms.

One can develop an order of acquisition according to sounds and sound classes. Not all phonemes of each class always appear exactly as grouped, but there is a general tendency for this to occur. The first groups of sounds that are customarily produced (not necessarily *mastered*) are the stops, the nasals, and the glides. Remember, though, that not *all* phonemes of each of these groups are customarily produced early. The second group of sounds, probably overlapping in time of development with other groups, is the liquids. These are followed by what some persons label as "more difficult" sounds (perhaps because they do require an older age, as that term suggests): the fricatives and the affricates.

Another way of examining speech-sound acquisition in broader groups is according to their positions in words. Some experts consider these positions to be the *initial* position, the *medial* position, and the *final* position. The speech-sound that commences a word is the initial-position sound, the one that completes the word is the final-position sound, and the one found in midword is the medial-position sound. (Some experts disagree with the idea of a medial position; they suggest that it might be the terminal sound, or the initial sound of a syllable within a word). Again, there is not a clear differentiation in this developmental sequence, only some generalizations: one expects the initial sounds to develop first; medial position sounds follow; and final consonants are mastered last. This sequence becomes less distinct in developmental acquisition stages in which some sounds are acquired in all three positions at about the same time, or when some sounds are mastered in one or two positions at one age, but at a later age in another position. It is important, however, to understand that there is a rather general developmental sequence according to phoneme position. What about the consonants individually? Are there any specific developmental acquisition steps that can be identified?

As noted in Table 3.4, norms are established for the skill-acquisition stages of

Table 3.4.   Developmental Emergence and Mastery of Consonants

AGE (YEARS/ MONTHS)	CONSONANTS CUSTOMARILY PRODUCED (+50% CORRECT)	CONSONANTS MASTERED (+90% CORRECT)
Before 2/0	p, b, m, n, w, h	
2/0	t, d, k, g, ŋ	
3/0	f, s, r, l, j	p, m, n, w, h
4/0	v, z, ʃ, tʃ, dʒ	b, d, k, g, f, j
5/0	θ, ð	
6/0		t, ŋ, r, l
7/0	ʒ	θ, ʃ, tʃ, dʒ, z
8/0		v, ð, s, ʒ

Adapted from Table 2.3, p. 31, in Stoel-Gammon, C., and C. Dunn (1985). *Normal and Disordered Phonology in Children.* Baltimore: University Park Press.

consonant production, both the 50% and the 90% ("customarily produced" and "mastered") levels. As you examine this developmental sequence, keep in mind that variation occurs among children. These variations can be numerically identified as a "standard" variation, or deviation. One does not expect phoneme acquisition of a certain consonant to occur suddenly on the day of the child's fourth birthday, of course. An age is given as a sort of average or mean, with full expectation that there is variation around that average. Let us examine some of the speech-sounds and some ages at which they are acquired.

Before the child reaches two years of age, he/she can be expected to have customarily produced (50% correct) such stop sounds as /p/ and /b/, such nasal sounds as /m/ and /n/, the fricative /h/ (sometimes identified as a glide), and the glide /w/. Remember that the youngster is exploring all kinds of utterances, including other sounds not fully mastered. At around the second birthday, the child will have added to the 50% correct level of acquisition such stop sounds as /t/, /d/, /k/, and /g/, as well as the nasal /ŋ/. Many of these sounds will become mastered in this period of time, but the 90% correct level or mastery of some sounds does not really occur for most children until the age of about three years. Certainly, up to this time, most children are developing speech that can be understood. The occurrence of inconsistencies (e.g., the 50% correct level) does not suggest that the youngster is not communicating.

> Although he has just reached his second birthday, Mark is very capable at getting almost anything he wants. He's probably spoiled. But, in terms of speech, when he's in the family car and has been there for a while, it's quite clear what he means when he gets very fidgety and not a little irritable and continues to repeat "toy-toy." A stop at a service station usually resolves the problem. One must remember that the meaning of the utterance, "toy-toy" in that particular context (long automobile drive, fidgety and irritable behavior, lapse of time since leaving home) might not be too difficult for a parent to guess.

The three-year-old child has mastery of the consonant phonemes /p/, /m/, /n/, /w/, and /h/. These are all sounds that at an earlier age were at the 50% correct level; now, with practice, feedback, and learning, they have been relatively fully acquired. The same three-year-old child will have added to the 50% correct level ("customarily produced") some new phonemes: the /f/, /s/, /r/, /l/, and /j/ sounds. Two fricatives have entered the vocabulary, at least a good deal of the time. Glides and liquids, /r/, /l/, and /j/, also become evident. This does not mean that the child will stop saying "wight" for "light." He/she has not yet gained mastery of the /l/; this will not occur until perhaps six years of age.

As the child approaches and reaches four years of age, more "difficult" sounds begin to appear in the 50% correct group. Among the new sounds are /v/, /z/, /ʃ/, and /tʃ/ and /dʒ/. These sounds are not mastered at this time. The sounds that a four-year-old may well have mastered (90% correct level) are many of those formerly at the 50% correct level: /b/, /d/, /k/, /g/, /f/, and /j/. This is a major enlargement of the speech-sound vocabulary and opens many doors for successful speech. (At the same time, the youngster's language development now is reaching fairly complex levels, commensurate with the phonologic development here reported.) Note also that combinations (clusters) of consonants, as in the word "play," begin to be mastered at about four years of age (see Table 3.5).

Although representing few phonologic gains, the fifth birthday brings truly major language development skills. The acquisition of language skills is nearly at the adult level. The phonologic level, being increased by perhaps as few as two phonemes, has reached a speech-sound complement level that is extremely useful in general communication. The two new sounds, at the 50% correct level, are the two *th* sounds, the voiced and unvoiced cognates. Our English vocabulary has a large number of words with those sounds, starting with "the" and "this" and "those," and having some skill with these words is quite helpful to the youngster now at kindergarten age.

Speech-sound acquisition still is not complete. In fact, it can continue on into the second and third grades. At six years of age, when our developing child is entering first grade, he/she now adds, at the 50% correct level, the /ʒ/ sound. This sound occurs infrequently in our language, in such words as "measure" and "treasure," and never as an initial sound. At the 90% correct level, or when consonant mastery has taken place, we can list /t/, /ŋ/, /r/, and /l/. It is at this time that we expect the child to utter correctly such words as "light" and "right," among others with the /r/ and /l/ phonemes.

> In comparing Betty with Marcia, one would notice among other things that they had very similar speech, especially in the use of consonant phonemes. Both would describe a lemon as "yewo" and a big jungle cat as a "wion." Sometimes the /w/ consonant would replace the /r/, in such words as "red" or "run." But in one the articulation was an important disorder, while in the other it would not even be considered different, let alone a disorder. Betty had a speech problem: she was eight years old. Marcia did not have a speech disorder—she was only four years old.

Our hypothetical youngster now moves toward seven years of age. He/she has completed going through the available complement of sounds and should not be using any at the 50% correct level. At seven years of age, he/she should have mastery over the voiceless /θ/ sounds, the /ʃ/, and affricates /tʃ/ and /dʒ/, as well as the /z/ phoneme. By the beginning of third grade we can expect even more development in consonant production. At the 90% correct level, the child now should have acquired the /v/, the voiced /ð/, the /s/, and the /ʒ/ phonemes. Final mastery of speech-sounds should take place by the time the child is ready for the third grade.

More remains in the area of phonologic development, of course. Perhaps little may be of immediate interest at this level of study, but a general comment to indicate additional development is in order. The acquisition of phoneme clusters occurs over time. Norms have also been developed for these. Phoneme clusters are combinations of consonants: the earliest acquired ones are /pl/, /br/, /tw/, /sm/ in initial positions, acquired at the age of about four years (Table 3.5). Some of the last to develop clusters, such speech-sounds as /kt/ and /sp/ in final positions, are acquired at about eight years. Having developed these consonant clusters, what remain are the phonologic areas within the melody, rate, and stress realms of speech development, until the full adult form of speech is gained.

Should an individual fail to demonstrate adequate or normal articulation skills, it is necessary to consider first the age, second the capabilities (adequacies), and third the nature of the phonetic (articulatory) error itself.

DISORDERS OF ARTICULATION

In Chapter 1 we defined a communication disorder. Adhering to this definition we can state that a person has an articulatory disorder when the production of speech-sounds attracts negative attention to those sounds, causes the speech to be less

Table 3.5.   Developmental Mastery (75% Correct) of Speech-Sound Clusters

AGE (YEARS/MONTHS)	INITIAL CLUSTERS	FINAL CLUSTERS
4/0	pl, bl, kl, gl	mp, mpt, mps, ŋk
	pr, br, tr, dr, kr	lp, lt, rm, rt, rk
	tw, kw	pt, ks
	sm, sn, sp, st, sk	ft
5/0	gr, fl, fr, str	lb, lf
		rd, rf, rn
6/0	skw	lk
		rb, rg, rθ, rdʒ, rst, rtʃ
		nt, nd, nθ
7/0	spl, spr, skr	sk, st, kst
	sl, sw	lθ, lz
		dʒd
8/0		kt, sp

Adapted from Templin, M. C. (1953). Norms on a screening test of articulation for ages three through eight. *Journal of Speech and Hearing Disorders* 18:323–331.

intelligible, and/or causes the speaker to be personally disturbed by the manner of producing those sounds. Of course, age level must be considered when applying such a definition. For example, one would not expect a three-year-old child to be saying /s/ sounds or affricates entirely correctly. Articulation disorders are not found only in children, so a definition must be broad enough to cover all possibilities. A vexing question in such definitions is how to consider geographic or ethnic speech differences.

In what ways can articulation be said to be disordered? How can phonemes be said to be in error? There are three, possibly four different ways this can occur: errors of distortion, substitution, and omission, and on occasion we may consider addition as another problem.

Distortion articulation errors are those causing the intended phoneme to be heard as something other than the intended sound, yet not as another speech-sound of the language. The distorted phone (the actual utterance that is heard) may be "something like" the model sound, may be "in the ball park," but is noticed because of its distortion. A common example is one of the several types of lisping, in which the /s/-type sound is produced by unusual constrictions and air flow, with audible turbulence quite different from the intended /s/. A lateral lisp is one that directs air flow over one or both sides of the tongue tip, not over the end. A protrusional lisp occurs when the tongue is placed between the upper and lower teeth (suggestive of the /θ/ sounds). Other distortions occur for other speech sounds as well, including the vowel sounds.

> The reader might remember the young boy in the movie (and musical) "The Music Man." This child was represented as having a lateral lisp. The reader may well have heard other children with lisps, especially the protrusional type in which the tongue tip is placed between the upper and lower incisor teeth and the resulting sound is a distorted /s/, perhaps seemingly close to a *th* sound. These and other articulation disorders occur with adults; some adults develop such problems as a result of changes in the articulators; loss of teeth, injury, or even dentures may be associated.

Substitution articulation errors are those in which another speech-sound is produced rather than the phoneme required in that situation. An example is the developing child's use of /w/ for /r/ or /l/, when he/she says "wun" for "run," or "wight" for "light." In the developing child, this could be viewed as age-appropriate even though it is not "correct." However, when this sort of phoneme substitution continues beyond the age range at which the child might be expected to have gained the appropriate skill, it is no longer acceptable as a developmental error. When this type of speech-sound substitution happens in the speech of an older child or that of an adult, it is an articulation disorder. There are a number of such types of errors, in vowels as well as in consonants.

> Some persons, such as Jeanne who has a hearing problem, substitute phonemes because of the way they hear words spoken. She hears the /ð/ as simply a /t/; so she says "wat" for "watch," and so on. Another illustration is the person whose first language is not English. Such a person may very likely substitute an /s/ for a /θ/, as in

"eser" rather than "either"; or perhaps substitute a /d/ to make "eder" rather than "either" or "dis" rather than "this."

Omission articulation errors are those in which the speech-sound required in a word is not uttered, it is omitted. Again, a commonly heard (but not disordered) speech example is the developing child's omission of phonemes: examples are "ca" for "cat," "wa" for "wash," and "tee" for "tree." Although acceptable in the speech of a very young child, such omissions classify as disorder types when occurring in the speech of an older child or adult.

When he moved from the Eastern to the Western United States, Leonard W. soon learned that his speech was sufficiently different from others that it caused attention to be focused on it. Among articulation differences ("errors"?) was his omission of final /r/-type sounds. In the East, he could say "caw" (or something akin to it) and people accepted it for "car" without hesitation. In the West, this did not prove to be the case. The question may arise: is this a speech disorder?

Addition articulation errors can be heard on occasion, and often are associated with regional (geographic) dialects of a language. In such a situation, it might not be called a disorder as long as most persons in that region speak in that fashion. Thus, the intrusive /ə/ (as in "cuhlock" for clock) may be acceptable in some geographic regions. Otherwise, and elsewhere, such an addition could be threatened with the label "disorder."

No one of these articulation disorders is necessarily the only problem an individual expresses. More than a single sound could be in error. A person could have different types of errors in his/her speech production. Often, however, there are patterns in speech-sound problems. The patterns may occur in groups of sounds, such as the fricatives, or may occur in certain other features such as place of constriction. Thus, tongue-tip (apical) sounds might be problems to one person. Also, an individual may have important problems with a particular speech-sound in some phonetic combinations, but have better success in others. It behooves the speech clinician to identify those situations, to find the phonetic environments in which the person does a better job of uttering the target sound. The clinician has then found an inroad into resolving the difficulty. The clinician must also take into consideration the reason that the individual has not gained complete mastery of speech-sound production. What might be some of the causes for the disorder? Knowing these etiologies provides another inroad into remediation.

Phonologic Disorders

It is important here to differentiate phonologic from articulation disorders. Phonologic disorders often appear to be the result of the child's efforts to "simplify" speech." For example, he/she might omit (not say) final consonants in whatever words are used. The youngster avoids a phonologic rule: all final consonants must be uttered. Or, such a disorder might be observed in a child who shortens consonant clusters, leaving out a necessary consonant (e.g., "clutter" for "cluster"), or eliminates syllables of words, among other phonologic errors. Such a disorder differs from an articulation disorder in that the child may well be capable of saying a certain consonant, for example, but leaves it out in certain word positions. Thus, a linguistic not an articulatory error is made.

Etiologies of Articulation Errors

In examining the causes of articulation errors, we need to examine capabilities, those prerequisites for adequate speech-sound development. One must identify the error sounds and study the speaker's age and capabilities so that appropriate remedial approaches may be utilized. Earlier in this chapter, five "capacities" were presented as those strongly related to articulation development. In a child with a disorder of articulation, a speech clinician should study these cognitive, sensory, anatomic, neuromotor, and environmental adequacies.

Cognitive adequacy suggests intelligence. Although intelligence is a multifaceted and tremendously complex aspect of our makeup, in the context of articulation skills it may be regarded as the ability of the individual to identify the target sound or the error sound as being different or distinguishable from another sound. Should the youngster or the older person have difficulty in making such discrimination because of intellectual deficits, then it might be understandable why he/she is not perfectly precise in articulatory skill. Children with cognitive problems (sometimes identified as mental retardation) may well be slower than other children in the development and stabilization of use of speech-sounds. Intelligence can be slightly or severely depressed, the degree being somewhat associated with articulatory (and other) skills.

Sensory adequacy primarily refers to audition but also includes other speech-related sensory capacities. It is important to realize that hearing plays an essential role in a child's learning to talk, to use the phonemes of his/her environmental language. A question asked early in an evaluation brings up the child's auditory abilities, or lack of them. In addition, other sensory capacities must be adequate. A decrease in sensitivity of the approximation or touching of articulators (e.g., tongue-tip to teeth) in speech-sound production, or in muscle behavior (kinesthesis), or in articulator posture or position (proprioception) may underlie articulatory errors. Auditory and tactile (and other) sensory input are important prerequisites to speech production.

Jeff is a 17-year-old who has had a moderately severe hearing loss since birth. Hearing aids and special education approaches have been of considerable assistance in both his communicative skills and his general education advancement. However, Jeff is clearly identifiable as having a speech production problem. Because he cannot clearly hear the sibilant sounds (among others) in speech, his own speech either omits or substitutes these sounds. For example, when he says the word "stop" or the word "watch," they may appear to the listener as "top" or "wat." Jeff has problems in other productive speech areas as well, including the prosodic component of phonology, that clearly identify his speech as different.

Anatomic adequacy refers to structure of the articulators and of the vocal tract. Lips, teeth, alveolar ridge, palate, and tongue are the leading articulators. Structural deficits in these may be associated with problems in speech-sound production. Dental problems are not commonly associated with articulation errors, but such an association is not entirely unknown. Tongue aberrations, such as tongue-tie or ankyloglossia (see Chapter 7), are known to be causally related to problems in the production of apical (tongue-tip) sounds. Palate deviations, especially cleft palate, are recognized as etiologic factors in articulation errors. The integrity of the vocal tract as represented by adequacy of the articulators is always examined by the speech clinician as a possible factor in a child's speech errors.

> The third grade class had two little boys, Mike and Roger, who demonstrated a similar omission articulation disorder. But, they had far different reasons or causes for their difficulties. Mike had had a cleft palate; he was born with the roof of his mouth open so that much of his air flow passed out of his nose. Roger, on the other hand, had a tongue-tie so severe he could not lift his tongue-tip to his upper front teeth. However, the boys had similar speech errors: neither could utter words with /t/ and /d/ or /s/ or /z/, among others. They certainly would not be managed in the same way, even though they had similar speech problems.

Neuromotor adequacy is another capability examined by the speech clinician in such persons. Malfunction of the brain and of the nerves and muscles responsible for the delicate movements of the articulators may cause the speech problems. Among the many types of disorders within the nervous system are those grouped under the term *cerebral palsy.* The type of articulation disorder stemming from such problems is often termed *dysarthria.* Dysarthria is a neuromotor articulation disorder. It can occur in varying degrees of severity in persons with certain of the neurologic disorders such as muscular dystrophy, myasthenia gravis, amyotrophic lateral sclerosis, and a host of others, some more commonly found in adults than children. Dysarthria also occurs in cases of brain injury resulting from automobile and industrial accidents, strokes, and other events that damage nerves as they course through the body to the muscles of articulation or to the area of the brain that initiates speech commands. Another neurogenic disorder is apraxia of speech, to be discussed in Chapter 5. A case history and special evaluation techniques often expose the neuromotor bases of some articulation problems. Chapter 5 explores neurogenic communication disorders in more depth and detail.

Environmental adequacy refers to the nature of the stimuli, the spoken language, as well as the encouragement and support surrounding the child learning to talk. An extreme example of lack of environmental stimuli is the rare instance in which a child may have been totally deprived of a linguistic environment. A similar deprivation occurs with the deaf child, of course. Other examples of environmental deprivation are those in which the developing child is not stimulated to talk, not encouraged to relate to others through speech, perhaps even punished in some way for such behavior. The lack of stimulation may be unintentional (as in the case of an isolated, otherwise normal child reared in a nonvocal speaking environment by nonspeaking adults who are deaf and use visible communication systems). Non-English-speaking parents can influence the development of articulatory skills in a child, but one must be extremely cautious in considering this a probable etiologic condition. Children so reared in this country usually come into frequent contact with American-English-speaking persons, in the neighborhood and soon in school settings, and this situation is not commonly associated with speech problems. Such a disclaimer does not mean that this cannot be a causal factor, however.

Two other etiologic categories remain. One is a multifactorial or multidimensional causal relationship. Illustrative of this combination of causes is the child with a neuromotor problem that also includes a sensory disorder. The child with some form of dysarthria may well display an important hearing problem. Such a child could also have less than normal cognitive capacities. In other words, a child who has not gained articulatory skill commensurate with his/her contemporaries might have several etiologic bases together. There is a long-time rule of thumb in the helping professions that applies to this possibility: when a disorder (or problem or defect) is found, always search for a possible second or third problem, and so on.

The final etiologic category is best identified as "unknown cause." Some specialists have their own terminology for this category; among the terms one might hear are "learned" or "functional." There may well be differences intended between and among such terms, and some authorities could have very specific intentions when using one or the other. However, our intention here is to suggest that there are very likely unknown reasons for a child to have difficulty acquiring skill in articulation other than those listed. More objective observation of the many children with these disorders of articulation will further delineate, define, and discriminate among the differing types of articulation disorders.

Thus, the child with an articulation disorder classified as functional may be seen by another expert who will term the problem a learned problem. In the first term, there is a hint that the child is simply *using* the articulatory apparatus differently and inappropriately to produce speech errors. The second term indicates that, for whatever reason, the child learned to utter phonemes incorrectly, and if a behavior is learned then it can be "unlearned," thus corrected. Neither is a satisfying or a specific term.

Identification of Articulation Disorders

Not all persons with speech disorders receive attention from specialists. Some simply do not know that such specialists exist. Others feel that seeking help only further spotlights them. Or, it may be considered too costly to seek help. Many persons with articulation problems are found, however. The processes of identifying the person, and then of examining or evaluating the problem, are varied.

In many instances, the finding process is performed by a family member. A mother reports that her son cannot say the name of his sister, Mary, but calls her "Mewwy," or he asks someone to turn on the "wight," at an age when she feels he should have gained mastery of the /r/ and /l/ phoneme. A wife notes that upon acquiring a new set of dentures, her husband lisps. A daughter notes that after her father's slight stroke he is having difficulty being understood as he talks; he knows what he wants to say but many words are unclear.

A classroom teacher is in an ideal situation to listen to the children in the classroom and to identify speech-sound errors. An employer eager to promote a particular person hesitates to do so, and draws attention to this, because of the employee's speech distortions. A drama director or coach rejects the application of an actor for a part in a play and ties the rejection to the applicant's unusual articulatory patterns.

Groups of persons are often screened by specialists to locate individuals with speech problems. In schools, speech clinicians often commence the school year with carefully prepared and administered screening programs. Large numbers of children can be checked by rather abbreviated articulation tests in such a screening program. Once a child is identified in this way, a follow-up and more thorough articulation evaluation are administered. Other screening approaches are conducted in college groups, or in the workplace by industry, especially in jobs requiring skill in speaking by the potential employee.

EVALUATION

Once a person has been identified as having a problem with speech-sound production, a more thorough evaluation or assessment of the disorder should be pursued. Such a procedure, though time-consuming and perhaps costly, is important for a number of reasons. First, a catalog of the speech errors must be made. The nature of the disorder can be explored and disclosed in a more thorough fashion, isolating important facets. For example, one should know not only that the child has a problem with /r/, but also whether the other glides are adequate. The relationship of the articulation errors to how well the person is being understood by others is important. And the client's own identification of, and concern about, his/her articulation problem should be explored.

A second purpose of detailed evaluation procedures is to identify speech contexts in which the client is more successful in producing the error sound. Special efforts are made during the evaluation process to explore this ability. The clinician assesses the ability of the person to be stimulated to improve articulation. This can prove most helpful in setting up initial therapeutic or management approaches.

Third, a detailed evaluation, when coupled with other data, provides information that might identify causal factors. Such information may lead to the development of management techniques to lessen or even eliminate disorder effects. For example, should a hearing loss be associated with articulation errors, remedial approaches can be taken (perhaps a hearing aid) that will facilitate subsequent remediation of the articulation disorder. An oral examination might not only expose an anatomic or physiologic basis, but point to the need for medical or dental attention.

Fourth, an evaluation conducted with care and detail can result in findings that exclude the need for speech therapy. Instead, the results may direct the client to other professional or clinical fields. For an articulation problem associated with a hearing loss, a first step is referral to a medical specialist (otologist) and to an audiologist for more thorough evaluations. Other findings could point to other specialists. Cognitive disorders leading to articulation problems might best be part of a total special education program. Neuromotor-based speech problems may involve neurologists, as well as physical and occupational therapists. It is entirely conceivable, then, that a careful and thorough articulation evaluation could lead to findings that such a disorder exists, but that its resolution lies in the expert hands of other specialists.

Many evaluation procedures are used. As one might expect, the procedure a clinician selects depends considerably upon his/her feeling of confidence in and experience with the procedure, what is known about its accuracy (validity), its cost, the time necessary to administer it, and what information it provides that will prove useful to the clinician. Various testing devices or instruments have been developed over the years and more will certainly continue to become available. The clinician, educated in analytic procedures used to assess tests of various types, selects the instrument best fitted to the situation.

Test *validity* refers to the ability of the procedure to assess what it is supposed to test. One would not use kitchen scales to measure the height of a table, for example, nor would one use an articulation test employing words that are beyond the client's vocabulary or are filled with other speech sounds that confuse the speech production. The other aspect, *reliability* of the test, indicates that the instrument produces the same (or similar) scores when repeated. One would expect the same kinds of responses each time, much as one would expect a yardstick always to indicate the same number of inches between two points in a measurement task.

Many such tests have been published. Clinicians may learn about these tests from mailed announcements advertising the products of companies producing the tests, and by reading professional journals in which researchers report their findings about particular instruments, perhaps in comparison with others already in use. Clinicians also attend professional meetings, at which there are usually commercial exhibits by the manufacturers and sellers of such tests, and they discuss evaluation approaches with other clinicians and observe their colleagues as they administer various tests. It is a dynamic, moving activity to remain informed about the various tests and instruments that are available.

Once the clinician has obtained sufficient information on the nature of the articulation disorder and its causal relationships, the remediation process can commence.

GENERAL MANAGEMENT APPROACHES

It should be quite apparent that remediation or management of articulation disorders is not a cookbook activity. One will not find a text that reports a method for resolving an articulation problem in which the child distorts the /s/ in a lisp or substitutes /w/ for /r/ (wabbit/rabbit), or in which a hard-of-hearing adult fails to use the /s/ sound in most of his/her words, and so on. On examining the capacities that are possible problem areas, one should quickly perceive that different approaches need to be utilized for different causal factors, even when the articulation errors may seem similar. One also notes that there are many different possible types of articulation errors, and they cannot be lumped together in a single approach. In short, one approaches remediation with a plan that considers the nature of the articulation error, the possible etiologic conditions, and the overall character of the individual and his/her ability to make changes.

As an illustration, a hard-of-hearing person with articulation errors might well use some form of amplification to assist in the remediation. A hearing aid or other amplification device could be of considerable assistance to this person. Another individual with a problem stemming from missing or abnormal dentition might need to have a dental specialist revise or correct dental problems before speech therapy can begin fruitfully. A person might need to learn that were he/she to elevate the tip of the tongue to somewhere behind the teeth and gently blow, he/she might produce a better /s/ sound. This is a placement approach. Yet another individual might have failed to identify the error sound as one he/she needs to produce; so, it could be of help for this person to develop auditory discrimination skills to focus upon the sound and its use in speech.

Once a sound has been learned in fairly narrow speech contexts, such as in a number of words or phrases, it is important to expand the person's use of that sound into everyday conversational speech, to generalize his/her command of the articulatory skill. This can involve the cooperation of other persons influential in the client's life. The mother or father can reinforce and reward the child's new speech skills. A classroom teacher may be similarly involved. A spouse or friend or even a college roommate may be called upon in the remediation process.

A number of philosophic approaches are used in articulation improvement. In the area of learning one hears of behavioral modification, operant conditioning, and other approaches that stem from studies of how people learn and how to utilize those findings in speech therapy. Different approaches are used in different schools, as well as in different countries. Also, one should expect changes to occur as new philosophies develop.

SUMMARY

Probably the most common of all communication disorders are articulation disorders. They occur not only in children as they develop speech, but in older individuals. The anatomic structures that are used to produce the various sounds of language are called articulators. The process of forming the phonemes themselves is articulation. Lack of conformity in producing speech-sounds is an articulation disorder. There are four types of errors: substitution, distortion, omission and addition. However, when a child "simplifies" speech production (for example, by omitting all final consonants or shortening clusters) we call the problem a phonologic disorder.

The normal aspects of articulation—what is commonplace or usually found— need to be considered. It is the norm that sets the standard and thus defines or describes the disordered speech. The study of normal speech-sounds is phonetics. Consonants and vowels are the segments that constitute normal articulation. These are categorized by the constrictions imposed by the articulators upon the vocal tract, by the effects this action has upon the nature of the resultant sound, and (in the case of consonants) whether voicing is part of the phoneme.

The infant begins building oral communication skills by learning to differentiate among the various speech-sounds. Having something to say, the infant moves into producing the various discriminated phonemes as utterances that carry some meaning. He/she learns to produce most of the vowel sounds of the language by about three years of age, but takes longer to develop skill in producing some of the consonants, the last one mastered perhaps as late as eight years of age. To pass through the sequence of speech-sound development, the child needs certain basic abilities, certain capacities. These include cognitive, sensory, anatomic, neuromotor, and environmental adequacies, as well as combinations of these and perhaps other skills as well. It is to these capacities that the speech pathologist looks when a youngster has not developed speech-sound production skill at an expected age level. These become etiologic conditions that dictate the complications in the case and the directions in which remediation should go.

A thorough evaluation of the speech and of the individual should uncover a detailed description of the nature of the speech disorder and indicate its sources. The clinician uses this evaluation to institute remediation or management approaches, or even to refer the person to other professionals for primary care procedures. Careful evaluation and recording of the individual's progress are made through the use of standardized tests and instruments.

As knowledge increases about the nature of articulation itself and the causes of disorders of articulation, and as new and better tests of evaluation and more effective remediation approaches are developed, our ability to improve the speech of persons with articulatory disorders progresses.

SUGGESTED READINGS

Prather, E. M., D. L. Hedrick, and C. A. Kern (1975). Articulation development in children aged two to four years. *Journal of Speech and Hearing Disorders* 40:179–191. *A presentation of developmental data, varying somewhat from Sander's (see below), in part because of different research techniques. This sequence has become popularly accepted.*

Sander, E. K. (1972). When are speech sounds learned? *Journal of Speech and Hearing Disorders* 37:55–63. *One of the most quoted sources of information pertaining to ages at which children can be expected to develop articulatory proficiency. Both the emergence and the mastery of speech sounds along the developmental continuum are presented.*

Stoel-Gammon, C., and C. Dunn (1985). *Normal and Disordered Phonology in Children.* Baltimore: University Park Press. *A thorough and carefully researched text concerned with the acquisition of speech-sounds by children.* Also see Stoel-Gammon, C. (1987). Phonological skills of 2-year olds. *Language, Speech and Hearing Services in Schools* 18 (4):323–329.

Templin, M., and F. Darley (1969). *The Templin-Darley Tests of Articulation,* 2nd ed. Iowa City: Bureau of Educational Research and Service, Division of Extension and University Services, University of Iowa. *A classic and thorough presentation of speech-sound acquisition, establishing norms and a standardized test that has been in use for a number of years.*

Tiffany, W. R., and J. A. Carrell (1977). *Phonetics: Theory and Practice,* 2nd ed. *The field of phonetics in exacting and detailed fashion presented in an authoritative and classic text. The book might be found in its first edition under the same title but with the author sequence reversed.*

Study Questions

1. If Johnny has a problem saying the /s/ in his sister Sally's name because his tongue is tied to the floor of his mouth, with what other speech sounds do you think he might have trouble? Do you think he could be taught to articulate better? What might be a wise action to take first?

2. Some people speak with air escaping through their nasal passages. If air necessary for producing speech-sounds is lost in this way, what kinds of articulation errors might develop?

3. It is important that you can distinguish "speech" from "language" in both normal processes and disorders of oral communication. Can you produce a clear-cut differentiation between the two?

4. If you were informed that a certain adult never used the /s/ sound in his/her speech, what types of questions might come to mind as you searched for a cause? Think in terms of the necessary prerequisites for normal articulation development as you work on this.

5. What group of sounds, classified according to "place of articulation," might be disturbed in a person who has lost the front portion (perhaps a third) of the tongue?

6. Phonation, sound produced at the vocal folds, is an essential "feature" of speech; if a person were deprived of this feature, what sounds might be disordered? Remember that there are two major groups of phonemes.

7. We said earlier that delayed language development is seen as language use that parallels the language skill of a younger individual. In development of articulation, can there be "delayed articulation" skill? In a child of eight years of age having such a delay, what might you expect to observe in articulation skill?

8. Would you expect infants in the prelingual period to produce any phonemes? What phonemes might you expect to hear at that age?

9. Describe babbling. Put it into the developmental sequence. What importance does it play in learning to talk?

10. If a person demonstrated an articulation disorder in one phoneme, would you expect a similar disorder in other phonemes? Give some examples.

4

Voice Disorders

Voice disorders are disorders of phonation and resonance. The voice is sound, of course, and for an understanding of voice one needs to have a basic grasp of the nature of sound itself, or of *acoustics*. The two dimensions of sound are *frequency* and *intensity*, or, as we hear and perceive sound, pitch and loudness. The scientific, objective study of the voice is the investigation of one kind of sound in all its dimensions and variations. The specific sound, voice, is produced by the vocal folds in the larynx in part because exhaled air from the lungs vibrates the muscularly adjoined vocal folds. It is necessary to understand not only what the vocal folds do but how the respiratory system acts to energize those folds. In studying voice disorders, then, we require a way to objectively describe the sound of the voice, the nature of the sound generator (the vocal folds), and the breath support system. Although not a subject of common discussion, voice problems themselves are quite common. Most stem from self-abuse of the voice-producing system, some from misuse, some from disease, and some from damage. Careful evaluation is important to determine the nature and causes of these disorders. From this stems one or another avenue of remediation.

In the following pages we present a discussion of *dysphonia*. It is defined as a problem of the voice as initiated at the vocal folds (e.g., pitch level too high or a breaking voice with a bad cold) or as a resonance problem (e.g., excessively nasal or strident phonation). This disorder of communication is also known as *voice* or *phonatory disorder*. Although thought to be a fairly common problem it is perhaps not often noticed, in part because we may not have a model of an "ideal voice" against which it can be measured.

To understand dysphonias, one must first have an understanding of the normal aspects of voice production. We will examine the basics of acoustics (physics of sound), of breathing for voice production, of pertinent anatomy and physiology of the phonatory system, and of the voice-resonating mechanisms. Since phonation is simply sound production, one must first grasp the rudiments of sound itself.

ACOUSTICS OF SPEECH

Sound is vibration in a medium. The medium we usually utilize is the air around us, composed of gas molecules. The vibration or oscillation of these molecules or particles in certain patterns is the essence of sound. Of course, in discussing human oral communication we refer to the sound that a person creates with the vocal folds. This sound travels as pressure waves through the air to the listener. Understanding the nature of sound is important to an understanding of both speech and hearing.

Particles of air (or of almost any medium) are set into vibratory motion by some sort of sound generator. Familiar things that vibrate and produce sound are the strings of a piano or guitar, the clapper of a doorbell, or a thinly stretched rubber band. These oscillating objects cause the air particles immediately adjacent to them to be displaced in a similar fashion. The vibrating air particles transmit their energies to adjacent particles, and these particles influence the next ones, with this transference continuing until the vibrating force in distant particles dies out. Sound in air cannot travel indefinitely, which is probably a very fortunate aspect of sound transmission.

Sound travels as a wave of pressure of vibrating particles disturbing adjacent particles into vibration. At sea level sound travels through air at a velocity of a little over 1100 feet (331 meters) per second. Although sound waves can pass through a variety of substances (e.g., water, walls of rooms), oral communication usually utilizes air-borne sound.

The sound wave has at least two basic dimensions. A sound is described in terms of the amount of energy propelling it and the rate (timing) of the vibrations that created it. A sound's force (or energy or pressure) is its *intensity*. Vocal intensity (or sound pressure) is a dimension that can be measured with an instrument such as a sound pressure meter. A sound pressure (or level) meter picks up sound waves at a microphone, processes the strong or weak components, and displays the relative intensity on a dial, a digital screen, or a paper record. This dimension, intensity, is a physical aspect of sound. It corollary in terms of the psychologic or perceptual domain is *loudness*. Although there may be a close relationship between the energy of the sound (intensity) and its loudness as the ear perceives it, that relationship is not exactly one-to-one. We describe the specific intensity of a sound by determining how many *decibels* (dB) the sound is above some reference intensity. This standard reference pressure is so small as to be barely heard under ideal listening conditions by the normal ear; it is called "zero" decibels. Some representative sound pressures that have been measured this way are shown in Table 4.1 for common environmental stimuli.

The second dimension noted above, the rate of vibration, is the *frequency* of the sound. It is usually described as the number of complete oscillations that the sound generator (a piano or guitar string, for example) makes in a second. Frequency is commonly measured in Hertz (Hz). The perceptual parallel of this acoustic characteristic is called *pitch*. In describing a voice, its lowest frequency is its *fundamental frequency*. Most complex sounds such as the voice show not only the fundamental but a number of higher frequencies (overtones or harmonics) as a part of the total sound. When an instrument produces a tone of a single frequency (a pure tone), its pitch might be judged as high if the frequency is high or as low if the frequency is low. However, most sounds in the world, including the voice, are made up of a large number of frequencies. The lowest frequency, the fundamental, is accompanied by a number of

Table 4.1. Environmental Sound Levels

DECIBELS (SPL)[a]	SOUND DESCRIPTION
5	Softest sound heard in quiet by typical, young ear
25	Country area at night
30	Soft whisper at 3 feet
50	Soft conversational speech at 3 feet
65	Normal conversational speech at 3 feet
80	Average city street noise from sidewalk
100	Person shouting at 3 feet
110–140	Amplified sound of rock group
125	Chain saw
145	Jet engine at take-off

Examples of typical sounds and their average sound pressure levels in decibels. The reference (0 dB) is close to the sound pressure of a 1000 Hz tone heard at threshold by experienced, normal listeners under ideal quiet conditions.
[a] SPL, sound pressure level.

higher frequencies. When the higher ones are in multiples of the lowest one (as when the fundamental is 100 Hz and the multiples are 200 Hz and 300 Hz, etc.), the sounds are said to be in harmonic relationship. When the relationship is not in such multiples, one might say that the product is not in harmony; it is dissonant, and may even be called noise! Frequency aspects are measured by instruments such as sound spectrographs that make paper records of the frequencies occurring in a sound, or by a "pitch" meter that produces a digital readout of the fundamental (or other) frequency.

Intensity and frequency, then, are the two basic dimensions of sound. In examining a person's voice it is important to start with these two dimensions. Using some type of instrument has an advantage over using only one's ear in that an instrument provides a quantitative measurement component. One can record these measurements in a file. Then, by repeating the measures, one can better determine what change has taken place with time or with treatment.

To repeat, we use various instruments to assess a person's vocal system. Some devices provide a complete analysis of the frequency characteristics. The sound spectrograph analyzes a short (several seconds) sample producing a graphic representation of most of the frequencies present in that sample and some indication of the intensity of each frequency. Another device provides an instantaneous report of the fundamental frequency in numerical digits on a screen. A pitch meter offers a single reference number that is often extremely useful. Other instruments provide more information, including not only the fundamental frequency but the tones occurring at higher frequencies above that basic level: the harmonics that are found as integral multiples of the fundamental tone. Most acoustic events (sounds) are complex tones made up of a fundamental frequency with its accompanying overtones (harmonics). When these frequencies are in the multiples noted, we speak of a periodic complex tone. Otherwise, in a random relationship, the tone is aperiodic.

A popular teacher, Ms. Zylstra, not only lectured with well thought-out ideas and facts but was pleasant to hear. Her voice had a fundamental frequency that was just right for her age and sex, and it had interesting variation or melody. The harmonics in her voice summed to a resonance quality that added to its pleasantness. Her vocal quality, then, added considerably to her communicative effectiveness.

These objective, quantitative measurements of the frequency characteristics are important to the assessment of a person's voice. One needs such data against which to measure the effectiveness of treatment procedures or of just the passing of time. However, such instruments are not always available to professionals who must make such assessments. Some are forced to utilize the oldest and perhaps the most unreliable of all instruments: their own ears. Perceptual judgments are fraught with problems, to be certain, but they may be all that is available. The value of experience in clinicians making such judgments is great.

Remember that voice production is important to oral communication. As noted above, the resonance or quality of the voice and its character are basic dimensions, and areas of disorders, of human speech. But one must not lose track of the fact that all vowels are voiced, that phonation must occur for their natural production. In addition, a large proportion of consonants require voicing or phonation, thus the phonatory component in speech becomes even more important. Furthermore, phonation elements are present in prosody: melody or intonation, stress, and the like. The importance of the voice itself in oral communication is quite impressive.

The energy with which a sound is created, its intensity, is the product of a force. In the case of a loudspeaker or a doorbell, it is partly the result of the electrical forces; in a piano string, it is the amplitude of vibration of the string imparted to it by a keyed hammer or by a finger plucking it. In the case of the human voice, the intensity is largely the force of the energizing exhaled air from the lungs. Thus, we have considerable control of the intensity aspect of voice.

BREATHING FOR VOICE PRODUCTION

The human respiratory system provides for an air exchange between the environmental air and the interior of the lungs (Fig. 4.1). Within the lungs, gaseous diffusion causes needed oxygen to enter the bloodstream and waste carbon dioxide to leave the bloodstream and enter the pulmonary air to be excreted from the body by exhalation. The priority demand is for these life-supporting activities, but voice production in the human is a serendipitous possibility. The air exchange for life processes is largely controlled by the central nervous system; the process is relatively automatic. The air exchange for speech purposes is under volitional control in the main; the human being in speaking can overcome central nervous system controls, as long as life processes are not jeopardized.

Air is inhaled by active muscular contractions that cause the thorax containing the lungs to enlarge its volume. This enlargement is in part the product of muscle groups that elevate the ribs. Because of the contour and the oblique orientation of the ribs, elevation is not only upward but outward; thoracic volume increases. This

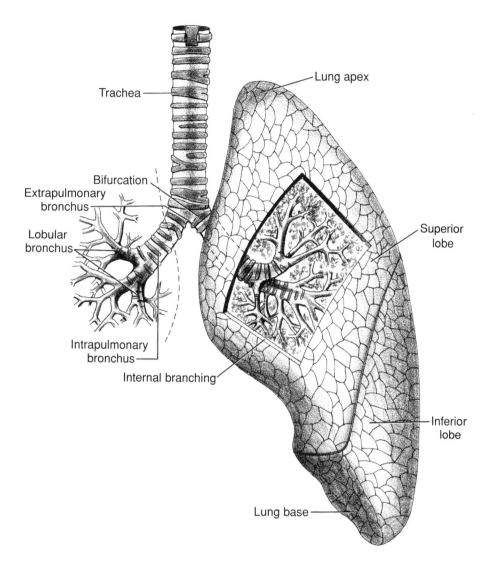

Figure 4.1. The Lung
From Palmer, J. M. (1984). *Anatomy for Speech and Hearing,* 3rd ed. New York: Harper & Row.

increase also results from lowering of the diaphragm muscle. In its resting position the diaphragm is a double-domed sheet that separates the contents of the thorax above from the contents of the abdomen below. Its muscular arrangement is such that when contraction takes place, the two domes, which protrude upward supporting the base of the lungs, are depressed and the vertical dimension of the thorax is enlarged. This enlarges the volume of the thorax. Thus, two possible active mechanisms, cause thoracic volume enlargement: rib cage elevation and diaphragm muscle depression. The muscles involved are under different motor nerve controls, providing a safety system in case of damage to one nerve arrangement.

Thoracic volume enlargement creates decreased air pressure within the thorax. This results in a difference between internal thoracic and external air pressure. At sea level, the environmental air pressure is slightly less than 15 pounds per square inch. Should the air pressure within the lungs be allowed to decrease below environmental air pressure, which happens when thoracic volume is increased, nature attempts to equalize the two pressures. Environmental air enters the airway and fills the lungs to the new thoracic volume capacity. Thus, inhalation is the product of air pressure differences, which in turn are created by active muscle forces enlarging the thorax.

Thoracic enlargement distorts the body arrangement, however. The ribs are elevated from their rest positions. Elasticity and other forces cause the ribs to return to those rest positions. In addition, the descending diaphragm muscle invades the abdomen and its nearly incompressible contents. The diaphragm is pushed back into its resting position as well, sometimes aided by the muscles of the abdominal wall to further force it up into the thorax. Rib elevation and diaphragm muscle depression result in thoracic volume increase, hence inhalation. Rib depression and diaphragm muscle elevation result in thoracic volume decrease, hence exhalation.

The elastic recoil of the ribs and of the diaphragm muscle is a passive activity allowed to occur by muscle relaxation. The return to the resting position causes the volume of the thorax to decrease, of course. Decrease of thoracic volume increases the pressure on the air within the lungs, which in turn expels the air from the body. The product is exhalation, generally a passive breathing process. In speech, a controlled relaxation provides for controlled air flow. This exhaled air flow becomes the source of energy ("subglottal air pressure") to the vocal folds so that phonation results from their vibrating activities in the airstream. Speech breathing, then, is somewhat different from breathing for vital purposes. It is under voluntary control, superimposed upon the controls of the central nervous system.

> Maureen at age 32 was found to have multiple sclerosis, a progressive degenerative condition of the central nervous system. It can be slowed but rarely can be stopped as it progresses. Among the problems Maureen displayed as she lost control of many muscles of her body was that of respiratory control. As a result, breath support for phonation (and thus resonance and articulation) was very weak. Phonation became shorter and shorter, so that she could utter only a few words at a time. And those few words were so low in intensity that they were very difficult for someone else to hear. Part of her communication disorder related to reduced nerve control of the respiratory system serving speech.

The exhaled air passes from the smallest spaces of the lungs outward (Fig. 4.1). It moves through the minute bronchioles into the larger bronchi, one bronchus exiting from each lung to join the midline trachea. The trachea, or windpipe, is formed by cartilaginous semirings interconnected in such a way that the tube is quite flexible. It passes upward, exiting from the thorax into the neck. Surmounting the trachea is the larynx, an enlarged structure of cartilages so formed and organized as to create a valving mechanism internally in the airway. The biologic function of the laryngeal valves is protective: to close the airway immediately upon entrance of a foreign object such as a crumb of bread or a drop of saliva. The valve prevents the object from moving further into the airway to reach the vulnerable lungs. In addition, the valve is very useful in that it traps inhaled air in the lower respiratory tract. When the valve is abruptly released, a cough or throat-clearing occurs. Trapping the air is also helpful when one lifts heavy objects or eliminates intestinal contents.

PHONATION

There are two sets of laryngeal valves; the lowermost set on each side is the *vocal folds.* They are so named because they are responsible for the production of voice, of phonation. They are the sound generators. The uppermost set of folds (*ventricular*) provides added protection, but is not commonly used for voice production. (See Figure 4.2 for general placement of the larynx in the vocal tract, and Figure 4.3 for an enlarged view of the larynx.)

The vocal folds create the vocal tone. They do so by setting up a wave of vibratory activity in the spaces above them. They oscillate, moving toward and away from the midline of the larynx as air is exhaled. The flow and pressure of the air serve to activate the vibratory behavior. Generally, the number of times per second that the folds vibrate becomes the *fundamental frequency* of the voice. The bursts of air that are allowed to pass between the vocal folds set the column of air above into vibration, and vocalization begins. Muscles within the larynx, as well as some attached to it from external points, cause the folds to move into the airstream; the force of the air then causes the folds to separate, in effect "blowing them apart." The muscles also cause changes in the contour of the folds so that they can be adjusted to produce different sounds, changing the fundamental frequency (or pitch), for example. The vocal tone that is produced is acoustically complex. Its wave composition is of a large number of overtones. These tones are carried into the chambers above where they are modified or resonated.

RESONANCE

The physical (acoustic) changes made in the original vocal tone are called resonance phenomena. The excitation of the air in the spaces above the larynx, in the pharynx and oral cavity, is created by the laryngeal tone. The nature of these chambers (volume, wall surfaces, coupling of cavity volumes) modifies the *harmonics* of the tone. Resonance is defined in terms of its effect upon an introduced sound. Resonance causes some frequencies to be selectively amplified (increasing the effective energy use) or damped (decreasing effective use). In more subjective terms, the chambers above the vocal folds cause the original vocal tone to have its characteristic *"quality."*

Resonance in itself is neither good nor bad. It is simply the modification of the original tone by the *pharynges,* nose, and mouth. (See Figure 4.4 for an illustration of

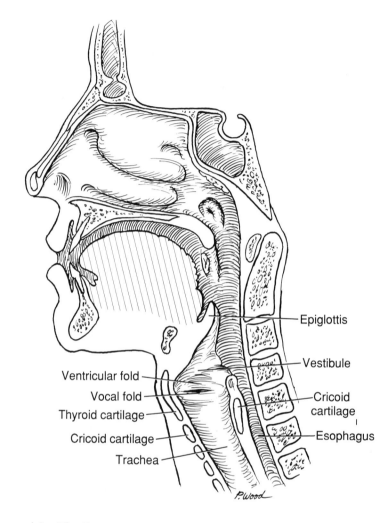

Figure 4.2. The Larynx
From Palmer, J. M. (1984). *Anatomy for Speech and Hearing,* 3rd ed. New York: Harper & Row.

these chambers as they fit into the entire vocal tract.) These cavities can be coupled to form one combined resonance chamber, or they can be separated to form single chambers. Further, each of the resonance chambers, and especially the pharynges and mouth, can be altered by voluntary muscle controls to change their volumes and their contours. Such changes would alter the resonance patterns, of course.

Illustrative of the resonance capabilities of chambers is that of common glass containers. An empty bottle can resonate a sound delivered into it. The size, shape, and wall texture dictate the resonance character (ignoring the nature of the original sound

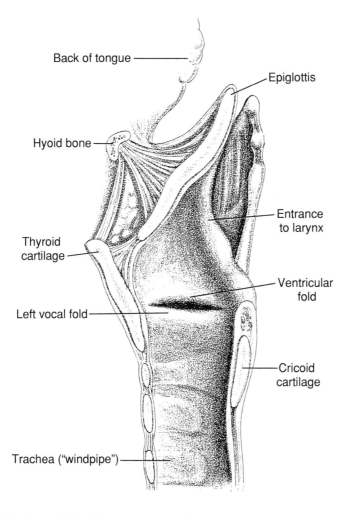

Back of tongue

Epiglottis

Hyoid bone

Entrance to larynx

Thyroid cartilage

Ventricular fold

Left vocal fold

Cricoid cartilage

Trachea ("windpipe")

Figure 4.3. One Half of the Larynx, Inside
From Palmer, J. M. (1984). *Anatomy for Speech and Hearing,* 3rd ed. New York: Harper & Row.

delivered into it). A large glass bottle resonates the same sound differently than does a small glass bottle. A glass bottle partly filled with water and then forced into vibration has a smaller volume of air to resonate, and thus a different resonant quality is produced than when it is empty. Variation of the quantity of fluid, and thus the quantity of available air, can create a difference in the resonance.

Vocal resonance can be changed in a similar manner. Creating a coupled cavity resonance by causing the vocal tone to enter the nose and the mouth at the same time brings into play another pharyngeal component as well as the extra (nasal) cavity. This

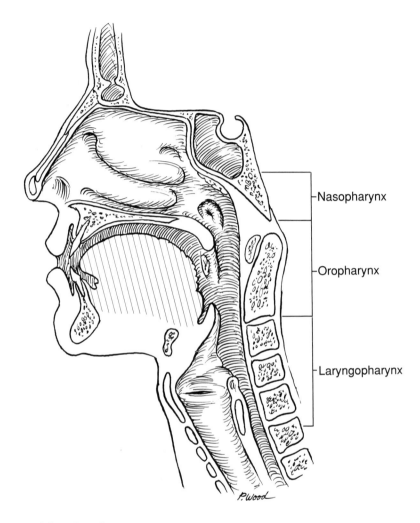

Figure 4.4.   The Pharynges
From Palmer, J. M. (1984). *Anatomy for Speech and Hearing*, 3rd ed. New York: Harper & Row.

is commonly known as "talking through one's nose," while a clinician would label it as hypernasal resonance. Vocal resonance can change as the result of other voluntary muscular activities, and of abnormalities in the vocal tract.

Mark was born with a cleft palate. The palate is both a bony partition and a muscular "door" that assists in closing off the nose from the mouth, in swallowing as well as in speech. Because Mark's palate was not fully formed, there was a fairly large opening between the nose and mouth. Not only did he have difficulty in keeping food from going into his nose, but air and sound for speech were also diverted into the nasal passages.

The loss of air for oral speech activities caused speech to be weakened; the shunting of phonated sound into the nose caused his vowels to sound "nasal."

Summary of Voice Production

The human voice is as individually characteristic as is the body that produces it. Differences in anatomy, physiology, and personality may be the bases of vocal variations from person to person.

The voice is the product of an anatomic system that serves the respiratory tract and a small part of the upper digestive tract. In speech production, exhaled air is the energy for phonation; a volitionally controlled relaxing and checking action develops a column of flowing air under pressure. This outgoing air provides the energy for the muscle-controlled vocal folds to vibrate and create a sound in the chambers above them. The nature of the original vocal tone, in terms of fundamental frequency, intensity, and frequency composition, is the product not only of the nature of the exhaled air but of the form and action of the vocal folds themselves.

The unmodified vocal tone delivered into the pharynges and other cavities above the larynx is resonated. The result is the vocal quality of that person's voice. The size, shape, wall texture, and joining of the chambers are the critical resonance effectors.

The voice is an acoustic event. It can be studied, measured, analyzed, and manipulated. Its fundamental frequency component is perceived as the *pitch* of one's voice. Its original vocal tone and its overtone wave composition form its spectral character; this is perceived as *vocal quality.* Its intensity component is heard as the *loudness* of the voice. When the system is disturbed by disease or by improper use, the person's voice may be unusual or disordered. The disorder is also known as dysphonia.

DISORDERS OF VOICE

Voice disorders are among the most common of all communication disorders. It would be difficult to prove this, however. Voice disorder does not appear to be a frequently used descriptive term or considered a "problem." To say that something is "common" suggests that someone has counted the "somethings." Counting voice disorders has been done only in selected populations—for example, in elementary-level school children in one school district. Prevalence studies have not been completed on an entire general population, such as everyone in Kansas or in Boston. Such studies would necessitate general agreement on the definition of voice disorders and the method used to identify the aberrant voice. In general, we are often uncertain in recognizing a voice problem when we hear one, so it is difficult to count the people who might have such disorders.

The very standards for "an ideal voice," let alone a normal voice, are not universal. What kind of voice is acceptable to you? What kind is not acceptable? Do you have aspirations to a "lovely" speaking voice? It appears that as a society we do not have common expectations for a "good" or "better" or "best" voice as we do for attractive hair, clear complexions, and other personal characteristics.

The identification of voice disorders is made more difficult because we use nonstandard and certainly unscientific terms to describe them. A host of adjectives are found in voice descriptions: hoarse, shrill, weak, thin, metallic, high, nasal, forced, and so on. Does each term mean the same thing to each person using that word? Is the descriptor meaningful and pertinent to the objective and quantitative aspects of voice: frequency, intensity, formant regions, air flow, air pressure, and so on? It often does not appear that way.

Voice disorders are important. To those persons who may have such problems, the vocal disorder may present a serious deterrent to vocational, social, or personal success. An individual in a field of work requiring considerable interpersonal communication, such as a salesperson, a minister, or a teacher, could be more effective if his/her voice were clear, pleasant, and attractive rather than hoarse, shrill, weak, or otherwise interfering with successful communication. Vocal problems are important to others as well: singers, children in school, even college students who "lose their voices" after attending a football game! Phonatory and resonance disorders may provide signs of disease such as cancer or neurologic abnormalities, or may be associated with important emotional problems.

Definition

A voice disorder, dysphonia, is a phonatory (laryngeal tone) production and/or resonance (quality) difference of sufficient degree to call attention to itself, interfere with communication, or create a negative self-perception on the part of the speaker.

Although they are not mutually exclusive, for purposes of discussion we may separate *phonatory* from *resonance* disorders. Disorders of (laryngeal, phonatory) tone include *breathiness, hoarseness, harshness, breaking* or *intermittency, pitch level* and *range,* as well as *aphonia. Loudness* disorders may be located at the vocal fold, or phonatory level, as well as in breath support or resonance chambers; as such they deserve discussion in terms beyond "phonatory" alone.

Resonance or quality disorders frequently are identified with overuse or underuse of the nasal pharynx and nasal passages as tonal resonance chambers. Thus, *hypernasality* and *hyponasality* are two common phenomena classified as voice disorders. Although difficult to separate from phonatory disorders, other vocal qualities may also be identified in this category; strident, shrill, metallic are a few of the descriptive terms associated with aberrant voice qualities.

Description of Types of Voice Disorders

Descriptive terms rather than quantitative measurement dimensions are generally used to identify voice disorders. The terms often refer to an audible vocal characteristic (such as high-pitch) and sometimes to an anatomic region (such as nasal or throaty). It is convenient, in the following discussion, to associate a general cause (such as excessive laryngeal tension) in some descriptions (such as tense voice), although causes will be discussed separately, and perhaps redundantly, in the following section. What are some of these descriptive classes of dysphonia?

A common descriptive term is *breathiness.* In phonation, this refers to the presence of audible air flowing through the larynx during speech. One might imitate it by commencing an exhalation with /h/, then moving into soft phonation while continuing to let air escape. A breathy vowel would result. Of course, one might have varying degrees of breathiness, from a very small amount to nearly total (*aphonia:* a complete loss of phonation). Breathiness is associated with the excessive escape of air during phonation.

> On the evening of the football game, Fred had a date with Anne to go to a movie and for a pizza later. He had no fun at all, nor did Anne. Fred could only whisper. He had yelled, shouted, and screamed throughout the afternoon's exciting football game. Then, of course, he "lost his voice." Temporary loss after excessive and abusive use had happened to him before, but never as severely as this time. He heard later that loss of voice has been known to become permanent, although not always just because of abusive behavior such as Fred's at the game. Since his educational goal was to become a classroom teacher, he reconsidered his priorities including his voice and its importance. He practiced better vocal hygiene thereafter.

One of the most common of all dysphonias is *hoarseness.* It usually develops from changes of the vocal folds, largely from vocal abuse. Hoarseness is described as combining breathiness with a hard glottal attack, or forcefulness in phonation. *Harshness* also has an effortful character to it, audible indications of tension. The laryngeal tone is aperiodic, and it also can demonstrate a hard glottal attack. Some common terms used to describe this voice are "grating" and "strident," although these (like so many descriptive terms for dysphonia) are subject to personal interpretation.

Another disorder is the *breaking* or *intermittency* of phonation. This refers to occasions of phonatory cessation at inappropriate moments while talking. It can occur rather severely, so that an entire syllable or a word is whispered before phonation returns. It can be so short-lived that it is a flickering of phonation, such as during a sustained vowel production. In the first case, when phonation disappears for a fairly large segment of speech, intelligibility can be diminished. In the second example, phonatory flickering, the effect on the listener is usually a qualitative one. The terms "phonation breaks" or "aphonic breaks" are sometimes applied to this quality.

At times, a person's phonation decreases in *pitch level* to an obvious extent. Of course, in normal speaking behaviors the voice lowers in pitch. One hears this in sadness, anger, or other emotional conditions. In the disordered voice with a consistently low-pitched phonation, it becomes obviously different. Is the vocal pitch too low for the age or the sex of the speaker?

The opposite characteristic, a pitch that is too high, also occurs as a voice disorder. Either males or females can have such a vocal problem, sometimes called *falsetto* when extremely high. Falsetto is the highest portion of the pitch range, commonly unused by the male. It is reached by the normal speaker through a pitch break at the uppermost region of the commonly used pitch range. A thin, squeaky, nonresonant vocal tone results. Attention is quickly attracted to an adult male using this pitch level. Again, is the vocal pitch appropriate to the age and sex of the speaker?

Another pitch disorder is *monopitch.* A speaker who talks at one pitch level, in the main, illustrates this. A professor giving an uninspiring lecture (at least uninspiring in its vocal characteristics), a minister showing apparent lack of enthusiasm, and a child responding to an accusation of an unacceptable behavior may be examples of a "Johnny One-Note." But a monopitch may accompany important anatomic, psychologic, or physiologic differences as well. A "monotonous speaker" may not be a healthy person.

> Both Joe and Mary had falsetto voices. Both were adults. Mary's voice was often mistaken for a child's voice. Listeners would glance quickly at her as she spoke, identify the person, and later remember her voice. Joe, on the other hand, had a falsetto voice that stopped any conversation, distracting the listener from what Joe had to say. His voice came much closer to meeting a definition of a communication disorder. It definitely interfered with communication, the intelligibility of his speech decreasing because of its high distractability level.

Loudness problems occur in voice disorders, too. In such cases a speaker uses vocal energy inappropriate to the communicative setting. For example, the person speaks so softly that the listener cannot hear or has trouble understanding him/her, or speaks so loudly that it offends or impinges too strongly upon the listener. On occasion, some speakers show problems of vocal loudness variation. Some have a mono-loudness, speech characteristically being too loud or too soft. Others may make words or phrases inappropriately loud or soft; they place a loudness stress on speech or language utterances that decreases intelligibility, the intention of the sentence.

Resonance problems in voice classify as *quality disorders.* For example, a voice may be overly nasal in its resonant character. As mentioned before, there are but three nasal sounds in English: /m/, /n/, and /ŋ/. All other sounds, especially vowels, should utilize predominantly oral resonance. When one commonly directs sound into the nasopharynx and nasal passages, coupling these regions with the mouth, the resulting nasal component creates another speech disorder: *hypernasality.* Too little nasal quality, as when one has a bad cold, is *hyponasality.*

> The speech pathologist was called to Rehabilitation Medicine Clinic to evaluate and help a teenaged girl, Betty. The girl had been injured in an automobile accident several months earlier. She suffered brain injury and had partially paralyzed limbs. Betty's speech, after six months, was extremely difficult to understand. The speech pathologist soon noted that it was severely hypernasal with accompanying escape of air through the nose while forming consonants. The problems came from the paralyzed soft palate that could not move into velopharyngeal closure during speech. Further study and testing determined that a prosthesis to lift the soft palate was helpful.

The extreme voice disorder is *aphonia.* This is a complete lack of laryngeal tone, of phonation. If the aphonic person wishes to talk, all that is heard is a whisper. Whispers do not carry far and are often low in intelligibility. For a person dependent upon speaking (e.g., a classroom teacher, a radio announcer, a salesperson) aphonia could present a seriously handicapping condition. "Mute" is a term colloquially used in such cases, although it has frequent accompanying misunderstandings.

We have described here a few of the various voice disorders, certainly the most common ones. It is important to know that the acoustic character of such disorders originates from some cause in the vocal tract. The causes may develop from aberrations in the respiratory system, since it serves as the power source for phonation, from differences in structure or function of the vocal folds, or from abnormal changes in the resonance chambers of the larynx, pharynx, or mouth. The causes may be associated with some combination of these etiologic events as well as with psychologic disorders and even some environmental influences.

Causes of Voice Disorders

Aphonia can result from disorders of the nervous system; damage to nerves serving the larynx may paralyze the muscles of phonation. Cancer of the larynx can also result in aphonia. Of course, the cancer is life-threatening and surgery may be undertaken for life-saving reasons. The surgical procedure, called a laryngectomy (meaning removal of the larynx), eliminates the voice-producing system. Not only is the person aphonic, but even a whisper is impossible. Some aphonias can be associated with emotional problems. In the past, the term used was "hysterical aphonia." Today, it is called functional aphonia. Emotional etiologies of aphonia include extremely frightening events, psychopathologies of longer duration, or emotional problems associated with body health conditions or pharmacologic agents affecting the psychologic health. Thus, aphonia is a condition with several possible etiologies.

Most of the remaining voice disorders are called *dysphonias.* As noted earlier, there is a variety of such problems and they may stem from a broad spectrum of causes. Perhaps the most common dysphonia is an intermittent, rough, breathy, perhaps low-pitched voice sometimes caused by *vocal nodules.* The voice is usually said to be *hoarse.*

Vocal nodules are small growths, benign *neoplasms,* on one or both vocal folds. The nodules are calluslike or cornlike growths. They affect the vibration of the vocal fold, and thus contribute to the hoarseness. Nodules usually originate from vocal abuse or misuse. By yelling, screaming, using improper singing techniques, loud talking over a long period of time, and other extreme vocal activities, damage is inflicted upon the sensitive vocal folds.

> Professor Lundeen was a vigorous and enthusiastic lecturer. His lectures carried to the back of his classroom, "loud and clear." Although youthful, he developed a condition that threatened his chosen work. At first, his voice came and went; but, as time passed, the condition lasted longer. Finally, the hoarse, rough voice became a permanent fixture, at times increasing in severity to the point of aphonia. Examination by a physician showed large vocal nodules on both vocal folds. Referral was made to a speech pathologist to remediate the causal vocal abuse. The professor learned to use better breath support, slower speech, clearer articulation—and amplification by loudspeakers to save his voice.

Vocal fold *polyps* are other growths on the vocal folds that may be due to vocal abuse. These are cystlike growths, softer and more malleable than nodules, but creating a similar effect upon vocal fold function. Phonation is often affected. Hoarseness, breathiness, and other phonatory aberrations can stem from polypoid growths in the larynx. Swollen, edematous vocal folds also may result from vocal abuse.

Another causal condition for dysphonia lies in the nervous system. The nerves to the muscles of the larynx are not easily available to injurious events, but such misfortunes do occur on occasion. Penetrating wounds or tumor growths can cut, destroy, or disturb a nerve en route to the laryngeal muscles. Such peripheral nerve damage may be rather easy to locate and identify. More complex are the upper or central nervous system disorders that lead to laryngeal nerve interference. These may be found in such diverse neurologic problems as parkinsonism, myasthenia gravis, multiple sclerosis, amyotrophic lateral sclerosis, and poliomyelitis. Identifying and treating such problems requires the services of the speech pathologist in conjunction with a neurologist, among others. As you might expect, caretakers ascribe first priority to life-endangering aspects and a lower priority to a speech disorder.

Dysphonia may result from other diseases of the body. Problems located in the respiratory tract, especially the upper portion, are known to cause voice problems. One of the more common is laryngitis, which refers to inflammation of the larynx. A number of conditions can lead to laryngitis, including some kind of microorganism such as a bacterium or virus, an allergy or allergy-like condition, a physical injury such as a blow, or some internally irritating substance. When there is inflammation, with or without infection, swelling, pain, and other effects usually occur. The swelling especially can create phonatory differences. It creates enlarged and irregular vocal fold margins, which in turn decrease the efficiency of the vibratory system for sound production.

Because the respiratory system, especially exhalation activities, provides the energizing force for vocal fold vibration, breathing problems could be causally related to voice disorders. Persons with health problems (e.g., myasthenia gravis) causing "shallow" respiratory quantities may demonstrate low-intensity phonation. Lowered loudness need not stem only from such problems, however. Extreme body fatigue, or health conditions that simulate this, also may affect vocal intensity. And, of course, emotional problems may be associated with loudness decrease.

In some dysphonias, a history of ingestion of foreign or unhealthy materials may be causally related to the vocal problem. One example, which is not at all comical, is the "whiskey voice." Some medications (for example, those given for thyroid gland disorders) may produce tissue changes in the vocal folds. Inadvertent or suicidal ingestion of caustics and other tissue-destroying materials can produce irreversible changes in the vocal mechanisms. Some of these ingested substances (e.g., alcohol, pharmaceuticals, or caustics) cause swelling of the mucous membrane, surface scarring, or muscle contraction problems. Evaluations of and treatment for many pathologies underlying dysphonia are usually done by the otolaryngologist, a board-certified physician specializing in ear, nose, and throat disorders.

As mentioned earlier, a well-known causal condition of dysphonia is that associated with cancer of the larynx. It occurs often enough that one of its effects, chronic hoarseness, is identified in public information forms as one of the seven primary "warning signs" of cancer. The American Cancer Society monitors cancer statistics thoroughly; its 1982 report estimates that there were some 10,000 *new* cases of laryngeal cancer in the United States in that year.

The vocal problem stemming from laryngeal cancer may be very real, but of course takes second place to the more vital aspect of the invasive cancer. Saving the patient's life comes first. Of several possible approaches (e.g., injected pharmaceutical chemicals or radiotherapy), one severe procedure is the surgical approach noted earlier: laryngectomy, removal of the larynx itself to rid the body of the cancerous tissues. In performing this procedure, of course, the phonatory mechanism is excised. Oxygen-bearing air enters the lungs through the exposed trachea in the lower neck region rather than through the nose, pharynges, and larynx.

> Ms. Clendon, who had smoked at least two packages of cigarettes a day for about 30 years, developed a chronic hoarseness that refused to disappear regardless of treatment. Finally, a laryngologist made a careful examination deep in the larynx and found suspicious growths. These, in laboratory analysis, proved to be malignant. To keep Ms. Clendon alive, it was necessary for the physician to remove her larynx. This included the vocal folds, of course. The result was that she became aphonic, mute, without voice. When she became well enough, a speech pathologist started working with Ms. Clendon and succeeded in teaching her to use esophageal speech fairly well. This technique uses a tiny bubble of air that is injected from the oral cavity into the esophagus where it is trapped, then squeezed back up to vibrate the esophageal membranes to create a sound. This sound is resonated and articulated as speech. Although not appearing to be "normal" speech, it did enable Ms. Clendon to communicate on the job and with her family.

Some voice disorders stem from emotional problems, ranging from the relatively mild deviations most generally healthy (emotionally) people demonstrate to rather outstanding disorders in severe psychopathic individuals. In the first case, for example, we can detect an emotional difference in a familiar person (e.g., a friend) when his/her voice is a flat monopitch, and we may conclude that the person is sad or unhappy. Or, at the opposite extreme, a high-pitched, melodic, fluctuating vocal quality may indicate a wonderfully happy person. In persons with important psychopathologies, these vocal qualities may extend over a long duration and become severe—even resulting in aphonia. Evaluation and treatment may well fall into the practice of a psychotherapist.

A last and interesting voice disorder is that associated with pubertal changes, as the child approaches adult physiologic status. Both male and female children move through this stage, the female's pitch lowering perhaps a note or two. The usual change for the male is nearly an octave in fundamental frequency. Most of the time most male youngsters pass through this changing time, because of vocal fold growth, with little evidence of change in the voice. However, at times (and not nearly as often as some humorists suggest) the growing adult retains his childlike voice or has difficulty sustaining his new adult, lowered pitch. Cracking and breaking pitch may be heard, much to the embarrassment of the speaker. Careful assessment is necessary to determine the immediately precipitating conditions—physiologic, emotional, or other—and thence to outline a plan for remediation.

Summary of Voice Disorders

Voice disorders range from complete loss of phonation (aphonia) to some form of voice problem (dysphonia) such as hoarseness, breathiness, harshness, hypernasality, etc. Because it is not "popular" to consider a person's voice pleasant or not pleasant, some voice disorders are ignored. There are no strong standards for normalcy, let alone beauty, in voice production. Many voice disorders arise from vocal abuse. Others may be associated with emotional problems, with infections or inflammations, with neoplasms such as cancer, and with a variety of other causal influences. Treatment certainly must have as its first priority the health and the life of the patient. Improved phonation, a better voice, usually follows. A careful evaluation must be made and appropriate remedial procedures applied to resolve dysphonias that interfere with productive life.

EVALUATION

At least two evaluation approaches should be used, if possible. One is the subjective approach, using the perceptual skills of trained observers incorporated with the opinions of persons important to the client, including the client himself/herself. A second approach is instrumental, developing objective and quantitative measurements of different aspects of voice production.

The individual assessing the voice should have some standard of normalcy with which to compare the client under study. That standard should derive from experience as well as an objective study of the voice. For example, the lowest (fundamental) frequency in a person's phonation might be interpreted as the "pitch level" of the voice. An estimate of such a pitch level, using the ear of the clinician as the arbiter, needs to be compared with what the clinician judges to be the standard pitch level for persons of like sex and age. Over the years, quasi-objective approaches have been used to estimate pitch level, using such assessments as *optimal pitch* and *habitual pitch* of a client, again in comparison with other similar persons, considering age and sex. Figure 4.5 illustrates normal pitch and fundamental frequency modes most commonly occurring for adult males, adult females, and children. Evaluation of a person's habitual pitch might be plotted on and compared with these curves.

Optimal and habitual pitch levels are derived from the individual's *pitch range.* A normal-speaking person should have a range of about two octaves singing up the "do-re-mi" scale. This may be somewhat generous, however, and a slightly smaller range is still acceptable. Recall that the lowest pitch should be the fundamental frequency, in agreement with the frequency of vocal fold vibration. One should look for the *habitual* pitch level. This is the most commonly used pitch level. If it is still normal, then this becomes the *optimum* pitch level, which should be about one-fourth of the way up the range (including falsetto) from the lowest pitch. The optimum pitch is the level we use with minimal effort or muscular energy. When an individual habitually

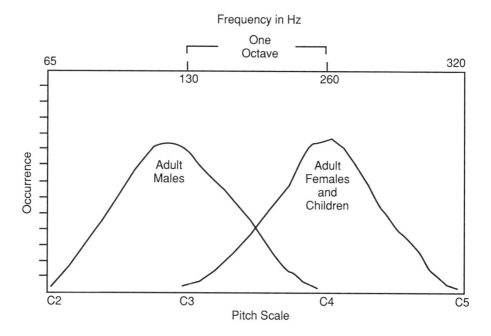

Figure 4.5. Ranges and Modes of Vocal Pitches and Fundamental Frequencies
Adapted from Fairbanks, C. (1960). *Voice and Articulation Drillbook,* 2nd ed. New York: Harper & Row.

uses a pitch level above or below optimum, this begins to qualify as a voice disorder. The popular text by Boone and McFarland (see Suggested Readings) provides several techniques and instruments used to assess pitch disorders, beyond the perceptual "too high," "too low," and "monopitch."

One might utilize subjective approaches estimating other characteristics of the voice of a client. The vocal intensity level can be studied as a loudness aspect, loudness being assessed in terms of its appropriateness for the situation. Or, one might investigate (again subjectively) the vocal quality and utilize a judgment scheme around overtones and harmonics of the person's voice as perceived by the listener. Tonal quality, including the presence or absence of the audible breath stream (a breathy voice), can be an aspect of perceptual evaluation. Other dimensions of the voice that might be observed subjectively include the melodic or intonation aspects of the voice, stress, and other observable characteristics. But the clinician's ear, as important as it is, is making such judgments on the basis of some comparison. The ear has some sort of standard against which it is comparing the voice under study. The questions arise: is there such a standard in every clinician's ear? And, do all clinician's ears have the same standard for comparison?

The various instrumental approaches to evaluating the human voice are partially freed of the weaknesses of subjectivity, except when it comes to the interpretation of the data. Some of the instruments used in voice analysis are acoustic analyzers. The fundamental frequency can be noted, can be tracked through speaking situations, and can be charted with considerable accuracy. The Kay "Visi Pitch" instrument is often used. The remainder of vocal production, the harmonics, can be identified and placed in relationship to the fundamental. For this graphic representation of most vocal frequency characteristics, a "sonograph" may be the instrument of choice. The intensity of the voice, in a single utterance or in a more conversational production, can be measured and charted. Various "sound level meters" have been employed to do this. Acoustic analyses can be performed by instruments in great detail or in somewhat general dimensions, depending upon the needs of the client and the clinician.

> It was not an exact time or date, but at some time Bob entered that developmental changing period associated with puberty. His body grew and changed, but his voice did not change. He retained a pitch level, an habitual pitch, that was not parallel to that of a normal adult male. Old friends were not too aware of this, but his new English teacher noted it immediately; he appeared to be "high-school-sized with grade-school speech." The school speech-language pathologist was consulted. Bob's habitual pitch was near C4 (about 260 Hz on the Visi Pitch instrument), or about an octave above what it should be. Her task was to search for possible anatomic or physiologic etiologies by having a physician examine Bob. No physical causes were found, and the speech-language pathologist turned to the task of habituating a modal pitch for Bob that was more appropriate for an adult male.

Aerodynamic measures can be made instrumentally. The flow and the pressure of air that are so important to the ultimate vocal characteristic can be studied. Flow rates and pressure measures may provide considerable information about the valving systems in the vocal tract. Such measures as respiratory capabilities using spirometers (or respirometers) of various types are sometimes used in further understanding the entire speech production system of a client. Breath support is an obviously related function, but may nevertheless be forgotten. Most dysphonia clinicians give it high priority in voice evaluation, however.

Other instruments evaluate vocal fold activity by studying transmitted light picked up after it has passed through the phonating larynx, or by studying ultrasound traces rebounding from the vocal fold margins during phonation. The larynx and the vocal folds are viewed optically and examined by fiberoptic endoscopes, laryngeal mirrors, or direct-viewing laryngoscopes. Most of these measures are recorded on paper, film, videocassettes, and evaluation judgments are reached about the vocal events. Such conclusions lead to hypotheses concerning the normalcy, or lack thereof, of the system. This information also serves as baseline data for follow-up measurements after remedial procedures (e.g., surgery or voice therapy).

It should be clear that the instrumental approach to voice analysis has many advantages over subjective approaches. However, because some instruments are quite costly and/or invasive, much voice assessment is performed without advantage of such relative objectivity. Only certain centers with fairly well-equipped laboratories might utilize such instruments. Some of the instruments currently available are not portable, but this disadvantage might well disappear in the near future as subminiaturization becomes more generalized.

No assessment is complete without a careful case history. One must seek for what may not be obvious: a severe injury, an infection, an emotional state, previous examination and remediation. What the speech-language pathologist identifies in the assessment must be placed in context with the information gathered from the case history.

The assessment findings, including the history information, may well leave a major doubt or question in the mind of the examiner. This may center on the health of the person with the voice disorder. Whether it is some general aspect such as a respiratory problem or discomfort in a body region or is focused in the larynx, this necessitates early referral to a medical practitioner (usually an otolaryngologist). This specialist seeks for problems with which he/she can deal, such as growths, paralyses, infections, or the myriad other health problems with which voice disorders may be associated.

A careful evaluation, however done, is critical in the management of any communication disorder. It establishes baseline characteristics, provides focus on the specific aspects of disorders, leads to notions of causality, and creates the rationale for means of remediation.

GENERAL MANAGEMENT APPROACHES

Treatment approaches vary. Why? First, the nature of the voice problems vary; second, the causes of the voice problems vary; and third, there are differences between and among clients (age, health, duration of problem, attitude toward problems, etc.). What are some of the general approaches that might be used, some of the more common techniques?

The first approach is to eliminate or reduce the potential for vocal abuse; recall that the most common dysphonia is hoarseness. The clinician may investigate the vocal habits of the client so as to remove the shouting, yelling, screaming, or other loud vocal productions often made. This may mean limiting the playground activities of the 12-year-old with vocal fold nodules, or calling a stop to his/her Little League sports activities. It may mean assisting a dysphonic kindergarten teacher in an open classroom situation to develop techniques that eliminate vocally abusive behaviors. It may mean guiding the minister, the salesperson, the riveter, the jet engine mechanic, or any other person whose occupation demands increased vocal effort, away from harmful vocal behaviors. Ridding the client of overly tense, loud, abusive behavior is a first step.

Some forms of vocal habits involve faulty tonal production. The singer utilizing vocal characteristics inappropriate to his/her vocal structures may need special coaching. Pitch levels, resonance changes, breath support, and loudness adjustments may be attacked separately or in concert in a treatment program.

Other forms of dysphonias that stem from anatomic or physiologic disorders may need special treatment approaches from the physician. In the case of a disease caused by a microorganism, an antibiotic might be prescribed and resolve the problem. Allergy treatments may be the only resolution in some cases. In others, surgical intervention may be the only avenue open, as in some cases of cancer. Surgery can be the elected option in removing vocal nodules or other growths on the vocal folds. Vocal nodules and some other growths can be surgically removed by, for example, "fold stripping." Voice therapy should follow to remove abusive behaviors that may recreate the growth.

> Reverend J. Finch was for years an extremely dynamic and effective preacher. His enthusiasm and energy and forcefulness could be heard throughout his church. At one point, however, these changed because his voice changed. At first, it would "crack," sound lower in pitch, and penetrate the church chambers less fully; close at hand it had a breathy quality. Then, one Sunday, he lost his voice. This clearly jeopardized his effectiveness in his work. On Monday, at his physician's office, he learned he had vocal nodules on both folds. On Wednesday, in a surgical procedure, the nodules were lanced free, stripped off the folds. The following Sunday he did not preach, but he carried on pastoral duties. In a few weeks, after returning gradually, he was back preaching as before. And the nodules returned. This time a speech pathologist taught him approaches to phonation that were not vocally abusive—and he lived and preached happily ever after.

On the other hand, in life-endangering pathologies such as cancer, the larynx may be excised (laryngectomy). Speech-language pathologists usually help patients following their laryngectomies. In some cases, the patient is taught to develop a new source of phonation by means of *esophageal speech*. Air is injected into the esophagus to be eructated voluntarily in a sound. There are several techniques for this procedure. Its product is often a monopitched sound with some limitations in duration of utterance. Some surgeons find that laryngectomees are good candidates for one of several surgical procedures that provide an air shunt from the residual trachea to the esophagus. This air is then utilized in sound production. Other surgeons who have performed something less than a total laryngectomy have inserted a valving system that can deliver exhaled air through what remains of the larynx. This may be useful for other than laryngeal cancer patients as well. Another approach to the aphonic laryngectomee is the use of one of several types of artificial larynges. Various companies manufacture battery-operated sound-producing devices that are hand-held and pressed against the external surface of the remaining vocal tract to convey a steady sound into the pharynx and mouth. This sound is then shaped by resonance and articulation maneuvers into speech. Another approach is the use of augmentative (nonvocal) instruments and methods: picture boards, computer-assisted speech devices, etc. These are discussed in Chapter 5.

There are other approaches to vocal rehabilitation. In some problems, an acceptable approach involves psychotherapy to deal with underlying emotional issues that may be contributing to the dysphonia. In other cases, metabolic (such as hormonal) changes result in vocal changes. Voice therapy is a dynamic approach, changing with the needs of the client as well as the nature of the dysphonia and its cause.

SUMMARY

Dysphonia, i.e., disorder of voice, is usually a perceptually identified aberration of the laryngeal tone and its resonated product. Instrumental means to identify and quantify the various aspects of voice are available, but sometimes costly, cumbersome, and narrowly focused in their measurement dimensions. The acoustic dimensions of the voice are the quantifiable frequency (and harmonic) and the intensity components. These have perceptual counterparts in pitch and loudness. The sound generator is the larynx, specifically its paired vocal folds. Muscular forces move the folds together in a phonatory posture, and subglottal air pressure and air flow from the lungs set the vocal folds into vibration. The vibratory rate of these folds establishes the fundamental frequency of the voice, and thus the habitual (perceptual) pitch of the voice. The resonance chambers of the vocal tract, the pharynges and the nasal and oral cavities, effect acoustic modifications (i.e., resonance) to create harmonic relationships that contribute to vocal quality.

Disorders of phonation may include abnormal laryngeal tone. This may be the result of deviant anatomy and/or physiology. Such deviations may be disease-initiated (laryngitis, cancer) or abuse-initiated (yelling, screaming, talking over noise). The laryngeal tone can deviate in pitch, loudness, breathiness, or other unusual characteristic. Resonance disorders may stem from the different use or nature of the resonance chambers; thus, vocal quality abnormalities can develop. Hypernasality results from failure to separate the nasal resonance chambers from the oral ones; or the vocal quality may be hoarse, harsh, metallic, or hyponasal, or other quality differences may occur.

Effective remediation stems from differential diagnosis, involving medical as well as speech analysis. Optical instruments, acoustic devices, historical study, personality assessment, laboratory analysis of tissues, the clinician's ear—all are among the battery of possible diagnostic tools to be used. Once the nature of the dysphonia is known and its probably etiology uncovered, treatment procedures may be instituted. These include pharmacologic agents, surgery, manipulation, ear and muscle training, and habituation reinforcement.

SUGGESTED READINGS

Boone, D. R., and S. McFarland (1988). *The Voice and Voice Therapy,* 4th ed. Englewood Cliffs, NJ: Prentice-Hall. *A popular text on the subject. Considerable detail of the nature of the disorders and extensive coverage of clinical (evaluative and therapeutic) techniques are provided; especially useful are the authors' "Facilitating Techniques" for voice therapy.*

Brodnitz, S. (1961). *Vocal Rehabilitation,* 2nd ed. American Academy of Ophthalmology and Otolaryngology. Rochester, MN: Whiting Press. *A classic dysphonia text with a strong medical orientation flavored by European approaches of long standing. It includes much consideration of the psychologic aspects of vocal problems. An interesting therapeutic approach based upon a vegetative chewing behavior is presented, which has met with some acceptance.*

Brodnitz, S. (1973). *Keep Your Voice Healthy.* Springfield, IL: Charles C Thomas. *An interesting self-help paperback book providing much information about the nature of the vocal mechanism and the voice itself, as well as many fascinating approaches to the care of both the voice and the larynx. Some approaches may not meet the test of scientific inquiry, however.*

Diedrich, W. M., and K. A. Youngstrom (1966). *Alaryngeal Speech.* Springfield, IL: Charles C Thomas. *An older text presenting the first instrumental approach to the understanding and treatment of the loss of the larynx from cancer. It includes excellent use of x-ray tracings in the evaluation and treatment approaches, as well as coverage (if somewhat dated) of means of developing a substitute voice for the laryngectomized patient.*

Green, M. C. L. (1972). *The Voice and Its Disorders,* 3rd ed. Philadelphia: J. B. Lippincott. *A popular text from England with a strong medical orientation. It covers both common and unusual dysphonias, including the abusive (hyperkinetic) types as well as "laryngeal palsy" and "inflammation, stenosis and benign neoplasms." It is a much-used text in many countries.*

Moncur, J. P., and P. Brackett (1974). *Modifying Vocal Behavior.* New York: Harper & Row. *A representative exposition of behavior modification approaches to rehabilitation programs. It covers in detail some aspects of behavior not focused upon by other texts, including relaxation and resonance changes.*

Prater, R. J., and R. W. Swift (1984). *Manual of Voice Therapy.* Boston: Little Brown & Co. *A practical text describing normal anatomy and physiology and including careful details of voice disorders, providing a description, causes, and management approaches for each in the same discussion. Specific management techniques and general health considerations are provided.*

Wilson, D. K. (1987). *Voice Problems of Children,* 3rd ed. Baltimore: Williams & Wilkins. *A carefully prepared and thorough discussion of the many vocal problems and their causes, evaluation, and therapies, including techniques for resonance problems and those stemming from hearing disorders.*

Study Questions

1. What does the text say about the differences among preschool children's voices in terms of pitch levels? Explain how you can distinguish the little boy from the little girl with only auditory clues.

2. In what two aerodynamic dimensions is exhaled air important to voice production, normal as well as disordered?

3. If one or both vocal folds are swollen, what effect might this condition have upon voice production? Explain the physiologic (movement) basis.

4. What kinds of health problems might create swollen vocal folds?

5. What types of behavior do some of your acquaintances exhibit that you might consider vocal abuse? If some do and some do not have voice problems, how might you explain the difference?

6. Explain in terms of the definition of communication disorder used in this text why dysphonia does not receive a lot of attention, publicly as well as clinically.

7. Define neoplasm. How does this term apply in the disorder of voice? Give two common examples.

8. If a person were a transexual, do you think that phonation might be a consideration in the process of changing? In what vocal dimensions might a difference be heard?

9. Would you be able, today, to examine visually the vocal folds? How do you imagine it could be done?

10. When a person loses his/her vocal folds, as in a laryngectomy, what might be the effect upon the functions of the nose? Think of all of the functions of the nose as you consider such problems.

11. Give some examples of individuals who might be seriously disabled in life (but perhaps not physically disabled) by dysphonia.

5

Neurogenic Speech and Language Disorders

Increasingly, speech pathologists are serving the communication and other needs of persons with disorders of the nervous system. As the general population ages, more persons with aging-related conditions will be seen. Another population served by speech pathologists is infants and children with known or suspected neurogenic communication disorders; in fact, laws dictate care for children aged "zero to three" and beyond. There are, of course, large numbers of other persons of all ages with damage to their nervous systems from disease, accidents, tumors, and so on.

It is important to get a general idea about the nature and function of the various components of the nervous system as well as representative communication disorders that might stem from abnormalities located therein. As you examine the normal aspects of the nervous system, you will quickly (and correctly) guess at the great variety of communication disorders and the possibilities for overlapping and combination disorders. We will first discuss the basics of nervous system anatomy: the central nervous system, the peripheral nervous system, centers and nuclei, pathways and nerves, and how they relate centrally and peripherally. Following this are descriptions of the dysarthrias and the aphasias (and several subdivisions of each)—speech disorders and language disorders, respectively. Assessment techniques and rehabilitation approaches, which vary according to the person and the disorder, are outlined.

INTRODUCTION

Speech and language disorders based on neurologic problems are rather common. Statistics concerning the prevalence for all ages are not well developed, although for some groups, especially the older members of our society, there are fairly adequate figures. At this time, it is estimated that nearly 20% of the United States population is aged 65 years or above. Every indication is that this percentage will increase over the next several decades: to 28.5% in 2000 and 35.4% by the year 2020 (*ASHA*, November 1983). Of the present population of persons aged 65 years and above, about 20% are reported as having speech and language disorders of some kind. About 43% of these persons say they have hearing disorders—a significant figure. In the area of neurogenic disorders, 2.7 million persons aged 20 years and above have a history of strokes (to be discussed later). Of persons in nursing homes, 19% have some form of neuromotor (dysarthric) disorder and 21% have voice disorders. Important here is the fairly large number of persons with nervous system injury resulting in a form of speech or language disorder. An even larger number have a hearing disorder, a matter to be discussed in Chapter 9. The possible or probable numbers of children demonstrating speech or language disorders are uncertain, but increasing attention is being paid to this population.

In this chapter, the subject is addressed according to etiologic significance. Other chapters focus on the acoustic or linguistic aspects of communication, but here attention is placed on those disorders stemming from a very unique causation: neurologic abnormality. Along with the communication problems encountered, other physical, physiologic, psychologic, and behavioral abnormalities may occur. To better understand neurogenic disorders of communication, one must have an elementary grasp of the normal nervous system as it relates to the oral communication process. A basic knowledge of the central nervous system and the peripheral nervous system is essential. While acknowledging the role of the autonomic nervous system, we make little reference here to the endocrine system, so critical to the normal physiology.

NORMAL ASPECTS OF THE NERVOUS SYSTEM

By definition, the *central nervous system* is the brain and the spinal cord, which form a single continuous structure that is housed within the strong bony protective shells of the cranium and the vertebrae. The central nervous system contains the *pathways* (tracts) for groups of nerve fibers passing from one center to another. The *centers* or *nuclei* that are thus interconnected (Fig. 5.1) make up another component of the system. We commonly consider two divisions: the *brain* and the *spinal cord* (Fig. 5.1). The central nervous system contains nerve fibers and nerve centers that receive incoming stimuli from other areas of the body, send commands out to peripheral body parts, and also provide for interconnecting centers and functional pathways among them.

The *peripheral nervous system* is composed of the neural elements that connect the central nervous system with other body areas. Thus, *sensory* or *afferent* neurons carry impulses of sensation from whatever part of the body their end organs serve. Fibers pass from the end organs through body tissues to enter the spinal cord or brain via *spinal* or *cranial* nerves. The outgoing nerve fibers, *motor* or *efferent* fibers, leave the central nervous system nuclei via cranial or spinal nerves, passing through the tissues to their destinations, usually muscles or glands.

The largest portion of the human brain is the *cerebrum*. It has two similar *hemispheres,* a *cortex,* and many centers and pathways (Fig. 5.2). The term "cortex" refers to the covering, the outermost layer of an organ or structure. The *cerebral cortex* is a vast accumulation of centers containing millions of synapses (where nerve

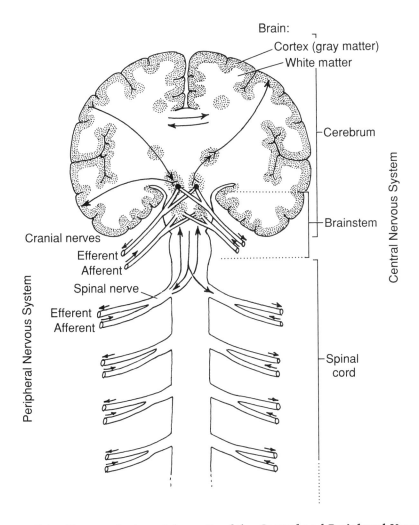

Figure 5.1. Nervous System: Schematic of the Central and Peripheral Nervous System

impulses pass from one nerve fiber to another). It constitutes part of the gray matter of the brain. These centers operate as principal functional areas. Some serve *sensory* functions, some serve *motor* activities, yet others are connecting centers. Major areas of the cerebrum and its cortex serve important functions related to cognition and memory as well as the very special functions associated with speech and language. Cognition and memory are important bases for human communication.

The *parietal lobe,* so named because it is housed within the covering of the parietal bone of the cranium, receives sensory impulses from the body in general. For

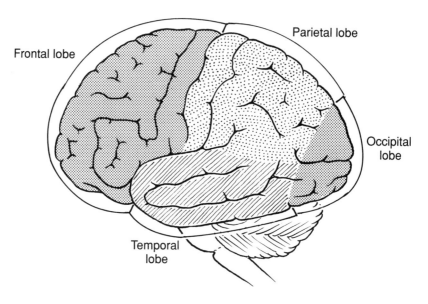

Figure 5.2.   The Brain: Cortical Lobes

example, sensations such as touch and pain are recorded in this region. The *occipital lobe,* similarly named because of its proximity to the occipital bone, serves visual sensations. The *temporal lobe* of the cerebral cortex, within the confines of the temporal bones, receives and processes auditory or hearing sensations (Fig. 5.2). The *frontal* lobe serves as the primary motor area (to the body's muscular system) as well as providing for memory, cognition, and personality features.

Nearly all kinds of sensation are served in one of three sensory cortical regions. Synapses process the impulses into meaningful concepts; further synaptic relays then take place to effect *perception.* Multiple connections among areas result in *association* regions. In association areas (motor as well as sensory), multiple inputs are combined to provide a multidimensional representation of an event. An illustration could be sensing a storm: a clap of thunder with lightning accompanied by a downpour of rain and a suddenly decreased temperature. The thunder is noted in the auditory center in the temporal lobe, the lightning in the visual center in the occipital lobe, and the wetness of the rain and the reduction in temperature in the somatosensory (body sensation) regions of the parietal lobe. The brain records the sensations, possibly initiates a reaction, and perhaps processes a linguistic label appropriate to the entire mélange of events. All are "filed" in memory to be recalled at such time when appropriate stimulation creates the associated environment.

Memory is a record in the anterior (frontal) portions of our brains of events and our reactions to them. As we analyze, classify, and otherwise process information, we use our thinking or cognitive skills. Our "brain-record files" become organized and we

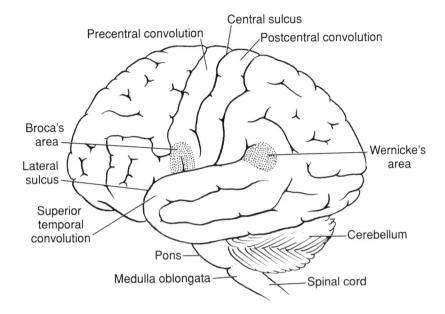

Central sulcus
Precentral convolution
Postcentral convolution
Broca's area
Lateral sulcus
Superior temporal convolution
Wernicke's area
Cerebellum
Pons
Medulla oblongata
Spinal cord

Figure 5.3. Important Speech and Language Areas in the Brain

codify activities. Our language areas place labels on events. The word "lightning," the word "thunder," and the word "rain" are linguistic (code) units representing the events themselves. The language area of the cerebral cortex (Fig. 5.3) is located posteriorly (toward the back of the brain) in the superior temporal gyrus. It is known as Wernicke's area. Note that it is next to the three major sensory areas earlier described. Here, codification takes place; thus the term "language area." In right-handed persons, it is usually in the left side of the cerebral cortex.

> Mr. Abercrombie suffered a stroke last July. An artery serving the brain ruptured; blood flowed out into surrounding brain tissue, destroying portions of the area. Thus, the brain lost the particular function served by that region. In Mr. Abercrombie's case, the brain damage was in Wernicke's area, the language center. He became aphasic, unable to call events or things by their labels, their names. Word finding was a very difficult if not impossible procedure. He claimed that he could think of the word; he could picture the thing or activity, but he simply could not say it. He had a language disorder secondary to a brain injury.

The cerebral cortex contains not only sensory reception and perception and association areas, but also motor centers of great importance. The synaptic relation-ships within the brain send the import of the received sensory information to motor areas for action, if action is deemed necessary by the brain as a whole.

The *primary motor areas* of the cortex initiate nerve impulses that ultimately reach muscles, and muscle contraction performs the task as planned in the appropriate brain centers. Below and slightly in front of the primary motor area is the *motor speech* (*Broca's*) area. In right-handed persons, this speech-programming region is found only on the left hemisphere. Damage in this location can place limitations upon speech behavior, even though the person may be aware of the words he/she wishes to use.

> When she had her "little stroke" at age 41, Mrs. Docent became aphasic. The aphasia lessened in severity over the months that followed, and about six months after her cerebral vascular accident, her speech problems occurred largely when she was excited or upset and her rate of speaking rose significantly. On such occasions, although she had regained her former vocabulary and her use of language was nearly as good as it was before her stroke, Mrs. Docent's articulation of phonemes became imprecise and her speech intelligibility level lowered. It was exasperating to say the least, for she knew exactly what she wanted to say, but "she kept tripping up on her tongue," as she put it. When she slowed or calmed down, she had much better control and improved speech.

The basic structural elements of the nervous system as a whole are the neuroglia and the neurons. In brief, the *neuroglia* forms the supporting, protective, and nutritive material in which are found the neurons, the functional elements. The neuroglia is found in both the brain and spinal cord. Several kinds of tumors may develop in the neuroglia, which negatively influence other central nervous system elements. This is a field of study in itself and is not of direct application in this chapter.

The other more active element of the nervous system with which we are concerned here is the *neuron*. This cell, with its cell body and fiber processes, carries nerve impulses. The neuron's functions are to receive and transmit stimuli along its fibers as they extend to and from its cell body. Nervous tissue is said to be irritable. The nerve impulse is an electrochemical change passing along the nerve cell fiber and across the synapse to be reinitiated as a new impulse in the next neuron or neurons.

As one might expect, the nature of stimuli varies greatly. A nerve impulse carries information about a sensation such as a pinprick on a fingertip or the sound of a doorbell, or transmits a stimulus to a muscle causing it to contract. It carries messages from center to center within the central nervous system. We stated above that the impulse is an electrochemical wave traveling along the length of the neuron's fibers; specifically, it is a wave of change in electrical (action) potential stemming from an exchange of sodium and potassium ions along the fiber (the "sodium-potassium pump").

A nerve impulse must be passed to a sequence of neurons. At the end of the neuron fiber, the electrochemical change traversing the fiber causes the release of a chemical (acetylcholine). This chemical stimulates the neuron next in line, or perhaps hundreds of such neurons. The nerve impulse passes from one neuron to others through the interposed fluid gap known as the *synapse* (Fig. 5.4). Again, synapses commonly take place in centers or nuclei—the gray matter of the nervous system.

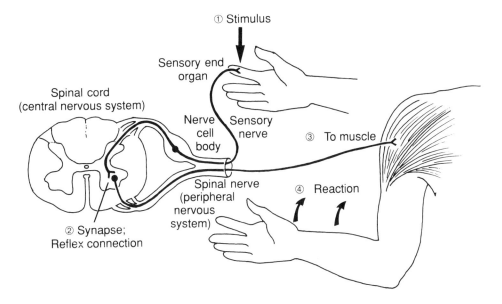

Figure 5.4. Neurons, Synapse, and Reflex Arc

The beginnings of sensory impulses are found at *sensory end organs* that are excited by individually discrete stimuli, e.g. sound or touch. These sensations are served by their own receptors; e.g., sound is served by auditory receptors.

Neurons transmit their nerve impulses (electrical action potentials) from one place to another via pathways or tracts, functioning chains of neurons and synapses. Hundreds of thousands of individual nerve fibers travel together. Outside the central nervous system these are termed "nerves," each named or numbered for identification purposes. Inside the central nervous system, the *pathways* formed by nerve fibers are also named or identified. As they pass through the spinal cord or brain, some neurons synapse along the way within various nuclei or centers. These nuclei are in turn functionally connected to a multitude of other centers.

The rapid jerk of a hand to avoid a pinprick is an illustration of a simple stimulus-response system, a *reflex arc* (Fig. 5.4). A receiving center records the stimulus, in terms of its source, its strength, and other characteristics. Synapses within the center may carry nerve impulses to muscles in reaction to an initial stimulus. Of course, impulses traveling from one center to another ultimately can effect more complex body reactions, perceptual awareness of the stimulus, or other complex neurologic activities beyond the reflex arc system.

A nerve impulse reaching a muscle sets off a chemical and electrical change that causes the muscle fiber, and the entire muscle itself, to contract. At the nerve and muscle fiber junction is the *neuromuscular end plate,* transferring the nerve impulse to the muscle. The functional tie between the two elements, neural and muscular, is again electrochemical.

> The diagnosis of Jerry's problem is muscular dystrophy. It is a disintegration of the neuromuscular end plates, according to some authorities. Without such end plates, of course, the muscle cannot be stimulated into action by the nerve impulses. As a result, the remaining muscle fibers that can be stimulated carry on the majority of the work required to perform muscle tasks, including talking. After a few minutes of talking or other activity, Jerry begins to fatigue from the effort. His breath support becomes weaker, and his vocal intensity less. Precision in articulation lessens because of muscle weakness. Speech becomes an effortful activity, tiring, and not satisfying to Jerry. As the dystrophy increases in its severity over time, the effortful and unsatisfying nature of speaking increases.

A large portion of the nervous system is devoted to *sensory* operations. The systems involved are termed *afferent;* they carry an impulse toward a central organ or area: the central nervous system. Our bodies are served by a variety of sensations, far more than the commonly identified "five senses." Two major divisions are the *near* and *distant* senses. The distant senses are vision, hearing, and smell; the stimulating event can occur some distance from the body. Near senses are taste, touch, warmth, cold, and pressure. Other internal sensations include awareness of position, muscle stretching, degree of lung inflation, blood pressure, and body acceleration. Diminution of one or more of these senses may have an effect upon the body's state, and perhaps upon the communication skill of that person.

Motor systems carry impulses away from a central organ or area: the central nervous system; they effect or create an action. These systems are also called *efferent.* They carry nerve impulses that may convey information to lower nuclei or activate muscle receptors. Centers in the brain and spinal cord act upon sensory information by stimulating (via a nerve) a muscle or muscle group to contract. The neural impulse may be volitional or involuntary, a conscious or an unconscious act. The brain encodes the action into an appropriate set of coordinated signals. These nerve impulses are distributed to the appropriate muscle groups to cause action in accordance with the original intention.

A large number of the speech and hearing nerves are *cranial nerves* (Table 5.1). The term "cranial" refers to that portion of the skull housing the brain. The 12 pairs of cranial nerves, in varying degrees, enter the brain with sensory information and leave the brain with motor (muscle) commands; some nerves do both, with certain portions being sensory and other portions motor. As is evident in Table 5.1, the cranial nerves most closely related to communication and communication disorders are nerves V, VII, VIII, IX, X, XI, and XII. (Note that cranial nerves are designated by Roman numerals and may also be known by their names.) Although the *spinal nerves* have input to speech (e.g., via respiration control), the cranial nerves receive considerably more study because of their larger speech and hearing functions.

Table 5.1. Cranial Nerves[a]

NERVE NUMBER	NERVE NAME	LIMITED NERVE FUNCTIONS[b]	
		SENSORY FUNCTIONS	MOTOR FUNCTIONS
I[c]	Olfactory	Olfaction (smell)	None
II[c]	Optic	Vision	None
III[c]	Oculomotor	None	Eye muscles
IV[c]	Trochlear	None	One eye muscle
V	Trigeminal	Head sensations (pain, tactile)	Mastication muscles
VI[c]	Abducens	None	One eye muscle
VII	Facial	Taste (gustation)	Facial muscles
VIII	Vestibulocochlear	Audition and equilibrium	Minimal
IX	Glossopharyngeal	Taste and gag	Swallow stimulation, pharynx
X	Vagus	Pharynx, larynx	Muscles of pharynx and larynx
XI	Accessory	None	Palate, pharynx, larynx muscles
XII	Hypoglossal	Minimal	Tongue and "strap" muscles

[a] Note that upper cervical (spinal) nerves may also serve the head region.
[b] Functions are simply stated and limited in coverage.
[c] Cranial nerves not commonly associated with speech or hearing functions.

Centers in the lowermost brain region control respiratory rates according to the body's need for oxygen. However, this region of Linda's brain has been damaged by a virus. One of her basic health problems is that she cannot control her respiratory rates. Secondarily, she cannot superimpose volitional control over an already disordered system to regulate exhaled air for speech. Thus, lack of air pressure for phonation and articulation decreases vocal and articulatory sound intensity. Linda is difficult to hear and understand.

One other subdivision of the entire nervous system is particularly specialized for involuntary reactions to body needs: the *autonomic nervous system.* It is entirely motor or efferent in function and is structurally a part of the peripheral nervous system. The autonomic nervous system acts without the conscious control of the individual—thus the description "automatic." For example, it serves to provide a body position change when a loud sound is received, to increase the flow of adrenalin in a frightening situation, to initiate digestive processes when food is taken in, and to cause the pupils to dilate in decreasing light intensity. The constancy of the internal environment, or homeostasis, is the general control objective of the autonomic nervous system. As such, it is not directly associated with those components tied in with communication and communication disorders. The autonomic system is associated with some body functions and malfunctions with which speech pathologists may deal; one example is dysphagia, a disorder of the swallowing system.

Summary of Normal Aspects

The brain serves speech and language, as well as its myriad other functions. The central nervous system areas in the cerebrum that are associated with intelligence, memory, and personality behaviors are essential to the formation of the ideas and concepts that the individual intends to communicate. These may be the products of internal stimuli (e.g., fear) as well as external stimuli (e.g., sound). The language region (Wernicke's area) of the brain reacts to codify the intentions into linguistic forms. These are further refined into speech productions by sequenced or programmed muscle activities, this refinement occurring in the motor region of the frontal lobe (Broca's area). From there and the primary motor cortex, the speech utterance becomes the product of neural impulses, with necessary neurologic checks and balances. The nerve impulses travel from higher cerebral centers to lower areas en route to speech musculature.

The musculature receives its neural impulses directly from the peripheral nervous system. Nerves arise in nuclei or centers in the lower brain and spinal cord. The centers in turn are under the control of the primary motor cortex and subcortical centers that have refined and coordinated the neural commands. The peripheral nerves exit the central nervous system, pass through canals in the skull, and traverse the intervening body tissues (connective, membranous, fatty, glandular) to reach the muscles they serve. Their nerve impulses cause muscle tissues to contract so that the desired speech act is performed. The activity is monitored by sensory systems to provide a correcting or modifying feedback system to the brain. This complex system can suffer injuries and disorders that ultimately affect oral communication.

NEUROGENIC DISORDERS OF SPEECH:

Dysarthrias

A number of speech disorders may be associated with damage to an individual's nervous system. Because "speech" refers to breath support, phonation, resonance, and articulation, the neurologic systems involved may be widespread and varied. Some of the primary sources of disruption lie in the motor systems, others in the sensory aspects of the neurologic control of speech, and yet others in association or coordination regions of the brain. Disturbed control of body systems necessary for life support may underlie a speech disorder. Motor speech disorders are often termed *dysarthrias,* some stemming from central damage and some from peripheral nervous system injuries.

Damage or injury to the speech-programming area can disturb the flow of speech. Speech can become effortful, awkward, or interrupted. In general, the fluency of speech can be disturbed by (1) impairment in just initiating speech; (2) difficulties in locating articulatory movements or placements; (3) hindrances in sequencing articulatory movements; and possibly (4) some language problems in grammatical sequencing. These occur even though auditory comprehension may be intact. They are frequently associated with problems in nonspeech muscular movements of the mouth or elsewhere. These four characteristic problems are commonly found in what has been called *Broca's aphasia.*

Among the dysarthrias are aberrant speech functions stemming from deficiencies in the respiratory tract. Breath support problems may be associated with respiratory cycling disturbances. (Inhalation should be followed in due course by controlled exhalation.) Examples of problems are found in some forms of *cerebral palsy,* a dysarthria in which motor control centers, modification areas, or relay centers fail to function normally in respiratory sequencing. The person may reverse his/her breathing cycle in the midst of a word or phrase. Phonation and speech in general are interrupted and disordered by such a nervous system disorder. Cerebral palsy is an injury (not a disease) of deep brain centers that may also underlie voice and articulation disorders.

Other dysarthrias may involve vocal fold function. Damage to the cranial nerve (*vagus,* or *cranial nerve X*) serving the muscles of the vocal folds can occur at its nucleus of origin in the lower portion of the brain or to the nerve as it courses through the body to reach the vocal fold area. Like other areas of the body, the larynx has a right set and a left set of muscles; each is served by its own vagus nerve. Damage to one of these nerves affects the vocal fold on that side. Complete severing or destructive action to the nerve causes paralysis to the muscles of the larynx that control vocal fold activity. The fold becomes immobile, and phonation becomes extremely weak, if not absent. A partial paralysis, a temporary paralysis, a localized or a generalized paralysis are all possible neurogenic bases for dysphonia.

One might identify a neurogenic voice problem in one of several ways. A very weak voice, one associated with breathiness or with intermittency of phonation, could be an example of a paresis (or partial paralysis). Or, as noted above, a complete absence of voice may occur; only a whisper may be possible. Such a speech disorder lasts as long as the underlying neuropathology lasts, unless some sort of remediation (such as surgical intervention) occurs.

Other neurologic problems are associated with dysphonia. Some, such as myasthenia gravis or myasthenia laryngis, or some of the degenerative neurologic problems often occurring in the geriatric population, are not seen only as phonatory problems because they affect other body processes as well. Although the voice aspect can be important because of its deleterious effects on oral communication, health care professionals might well focus on the broader problems first.

The dysarthrias are exemplified also by vocal quality and resonance problems. The muscles of the pharynx and the soft palate can be paretic or paralyzed. Probably the main source of resonance problems is defective velopharyngeal closure. When this is disturbed by neurologic events, coupled cavity resonance can occur, which is perceived as hypernasality. Acoustic energies are delivered into both the nasopharynx and nasal passages, adding an overly nasal (hypernasal) quality to the voice.

Articulation problems also may arise from failure of velopharyngeal closure. The air flow and pressure from exhaled air escape into the nasopharynx and beyond. This air cannot be used in the oral production of phonemes. Stops, fricatives, and affricates are to a large extent aerodynamic sounds. If the desired oral air flow and pressure are "bled off" elsewhere before reaching the mouth, the phones will be weakened or omitted. Usually the effect is weakening, but in severe cases it becomes omission of the phoneme. And the nasal air escape may even be audible in its turbulent passage through the nose.

> Jim had been able to buy a motorcycle when he was just past his 23rd birthday. It provided transportation to his work and a great deal of enjoyment. It also provided him with a serious brain injury when it skidded on a slippery street and bounced off a curb into a truck. Jim's recovery was only fair in that he had a severe weakness on one side of his body and visual problems, and his speech was hypernasal and very indistinct. Although he became physically able to return to some activities, including limited work, he was advised not to do so because of his poorly intelligible speech. Later, a plastic device attached to his teeth was fitted by a prosthodontist with the assistance of a speech pathologist. This palatal lift reached back toward his pharynx, lifted his soft palate and held it up. As Jim developed accommodation to the prosthesis, his speech pathologist helped him to decrease the effects of the palatal weakness. Speech intelligibility increased significantly.

Other neurogenic speech disorders (dysarthrias), especially those in the realm of articulation, may occur with damage to other nerves serving the speech activity. The muscles around the mouth that are important for lip sounds are served by the *facial nerve (cranial nerve VII)*. Damage to this nerve on one side could lessen slightly the effectiveness of the lips in producing /p/, /b/, /f/, and /v/ sounds. The *hypoglossal nerve (cranial nerve XII)* supplies the muscles of the tongue. When this nerve is cut or injured, the result would be disturbed movements of the tongue (the primary articulator) in attempts to produce many vowels and consonants.

As noted earlier, cerebral palsy is a brain injury that displays its effects upon all aspects of speech as well as other body functions and activities. The several forms of this disorder may differ considerably, in part because of differences in the brain injury. Thanks to the efforts of the United Cerebral Palsy organization there is now a better public understanding of the nature of the problem. Developments include rehabilitation and residency centers, special educational programs, and laws and facilities (e.g., handicapped parking, public buses with special devices) to ease the limitations upon these people. The brain injury commonly occurs in the perinatal period (around the time of birth). Many devices and instruments have been developed to assist persons with cerebral palsy to compensate for their various disorders; today one frequently sees motorized wheelchairs, computer-assisted communication equipment, and other assistive devices. This neurogenic disorder may not be "curable," but there are numerous ways to improve the lives of those having the problem.

> Mary Beth was identified at birth as having a spastic form of cerebral palsy. It probably developed during the gestation period because of certain blood chemistry problems;

the result was damage to brain centers below the cerebral cortex that controlled coordinated (and especially inhibitory) nerve impulses to the muscles of Mary Beth's body. The effects included major leg muscle (walking) problems, trunk muscle (posture) differences, arm muscle control (feeding) defects, and as you might expect, speech musculature control deficiencies that led to an important speech disorder.

These few illustrations should indicate that speech may be affected by abnormalities within the nervous system serving the speech musculature. The activities of breath support, phonation, resonance, and articulation are included among the possible areas for disturbance. When such speech problems derive from neurologic injury, they are often classified as the dysarthrias.

Apraxia of Speech

Another disorder of neurologic origin is *apraxia of speech.* Apraxia (or dyspraxia) is frequently described as an inability to execute purposeful movements in the absence of paralysis, sometimes due to a defect in cortical integration. "Purposeful movements" are those that are consciously performed. Speech is considered such an activity. On the other hand, of course, the speech mechanisms are used for basic life-supporting functions as well. Chewing and swallowing are good examples of behaviors that need not be consciously performed. Thus, an apraxic (or dyspraxic) individual might have no eating problems but considerable difficulty using the same body systems for speech purposes. Apraxia of speech often results in speech-sound distortions, substitutions, and prosodic alterations of inconsistent nature and occurrence.

Having recovered sufficiently from her neurologic damage, Ms. Fitch returned to her home to convalesce. She could care for herself fairly well and entertained herself by reading and watching television. Her communication problem became evident when she spoke. She would talk about reading a "fook—no, a b-b-book" or she would report on seeing an event on "lelevision." Ms. Fitch was quickly aware, usually, of her errors. She would self-correct, to some extent. But, she became very careful in speaking. She'd plan what she wanted to say, often avoiding words she felt difficult. Her rate of speech decreased because of her efforts. She repeated sounds and words, very much as stutterers do. Yet, she always knew what she wanted to say. And, she knew when she erred. She could not control the mechanisms to produce the speech to express what she wanted to say.

Experts consider apraxia of speech to stem from faulty programming of articulator movement patterns. Voluntary control of those muscles required for speech production often becomes disordered when the left cerebral hemisphere is injured. The speaker may be aware of what he/she wishes to say; the *intention* to speak is intact to the extent that there is a plan for the phonologic nature of the utterance. However, the speaker is unable to translate that plan into coordinated patterns of articulatory movements for speech. The disorder is specific to speech itself; the musculature otherwise does not show any significant weakness, slowness, or incoordination when used for reflexive or automatic activities. However, in some more severe cases the problem may occur as an oral apraxia, extending beyond speech production.

NEUROGENIC DISORDERS OF LANGUAGE

Types of Disorders

The *language* disorders of oral communication stemming from neurologic defects or abnormalities are several. Common among these are the *aphasias,* defined as disorders in the use of language usually stemming from injury to the left side of the brain. Here the disorder may be in the reception, perception, and recall of language as well as in language formulation and expression. In addition to oral communication, aphasia problems might include reading, writing, and other symbolic skills. Thus the aphasias are language disorders, in contrast to the dysarthrias which are speech disorders. One should not be surprised to find both general disorder types in the same disabled person, however.

Receptive dysphasia is a type of language disorder caused by brain injury or degeneration. What is lost is the understanding of words, sentences, and intentions of speakers; thus, one finds semantic, syntactic, and pragmatic confusions (see Chapter 2). Language reception may be disturbed in modalities other than oral communication—reading, for example. A receptive language problem can be very serious for it not only disturbs a person's abilities to understand a speaker's message, but also interferes with the aphasic's own expressive language. It deters the speaker's ability to monitor his/her own speech: not hearing the mistakes, he/she does not correct them.

On the other hand, *expressive* language disorders need not be attributable only to receptive diminution. Brain damage may affect areas responsible for the formulation of language. Inabilities to find the appropriate word, to form an intelligible grammatical expression, or to place utterances in proper tenses are some expressive language problems one might find in aphasia. Of these, word-finding problems are the most universal.

> Mr. Black suffered a stroke about a year ago and retains some vestiges of the original problem. One disorder he has is a paralysis of the right side of his body, thus keeping him from his work and his usual hobbies and interests. Another serious problem that remains is in his oral communication. He seems to know what he wants to say, but the wrong word or a strange word or phrase may be uttered. For example, at dinner he may ask his wife to pass "the spoon" when his intention is to get the butter. Mr. Black knows immediately that he did not say what he intended, and with some effort says, "No, no, not 'spoon' . . . " and with emphasis, "I mean—SPOON! No, you know—that stuff there" pointing to the butter. He becomes upset not only because of his original error but because he repeated the same error when he tried to correct it.

Aphasia, then, can be identified in several language uses: expressive, receptive, combinations of these two, language processing, and memory. It can also occur in varying degrees of severity from very mild with only occasional "slips" to extremely severe. The latter is demonstrated in an individual having no residual observable language functions; a disorder of this extreme severity is considered "global." The causes of such variations lie in the individual and in the different ways and degrees in which persons can suffer brain injury.

Special Types of Aphasia

The illustrations above represent but a few of the several types of aphasia. With different authorities studying and classifying the disorders, one might expect differences in their classification, labeling, and terminology as time and research continue. Some of the more commonly accepted types are listed, briefly described, and illustrated in the following paragraphs. Specific and detailed characteristics are not provided and may be found in specialized texts.

Recall that Broca's aphasia, a nonfluent type usually classified as a speech disorder, may include a language component. It can be listed as a language aphasia or simply identified as one of the several aphasia types. But it is more commonly assumed to be a largely motor speech disorder. On the other hand, the more fluent aphasias can be considered primarily language-focused. (Of course, they may include a motor speech component as well.) Patients with these disorders display fluent or flowing speech, perhaps retaining articulatory and prosodic skills. One might hear such a speaker producing a series of words, but the phrase may carry no understandable message. The utterances lack grammatical glue. And they might be words entirely inappropriate for the situation.

> Mrs. Falston, a pleasant 64-year-old widow, has made maximum physical recovery from her stroke 18 months ago. She is proving to be very difficult to care for, her daughter reports, for not only is she nearly impossible to understand but she fails to grasp simple requests and directions spoken to her. She does not follow television story lines and cannot watch television for long with any pleasure. She does seem to like to talk, however, even if it is difficult to understand what she has to say. A visitor entered her living room the other day, gave her a hug, and made a gracious comment about Mrs. Falston's dress, asking when and where she bought it. Her response: "Why it's fine but washed in the day-to-day cooking even when the sun is shining although I did find them after the door was opened when Myrtle was washing the dishes . . . ," and perhaps she could have continued indefinitely.

The preceding illustration might represent *Wernicke's aphasia.* It is sometimes called "syntactic" aphasia. The patient's spoken language may be fluent and well-articulated. The words, however, do not coalesce to make a grammatically proper message. This is the most common of the fluent aphasias. There is a common word-finding problem. It may well stem from an underlying difficulty in auditory monitoring and association. The patient with Wernicke's aphasia not only may fail to grasp fully what other people are saying, but by the same means (or lack of means) fails to monitor and associate his/her own spoken language. The patient is unaware that what he/she intended to say is not what was actually said. Such communication disorders may stem from injury to the posterior portion of the left auditory cortex, where auditory associations are made.

Another fluent aphasia is *anomia*. It is sometimes called "semantic" aphasia or "nominal" aphasia. The patient demonstrates word-finding difficulties; substantive words especially seem to be troublesome. In such a situation, a patient often engages in circumlocution (describes the missing word without using it). This, as in all the aphasias, can be a disorder of minimal degree or can be a major and serious problem.

> Two of the aphasic patients in the clinic waiting room are Mr. Reid and Ms. Schneider. His problem is classified as syntactic aphasia. Hers is semantic aphasia, both of moderate degree. When approaching the waiting room, one can hear Mr. Reid chatting vigorously with Ms. Schneider, but seldom does she respond. From a little distance, and being unable to pick out words, one judges Mr. Reid's voice as normal, sounding pretty much like everyday talking. On approaching closer and listening more attentively, one hears " . . . cut with a fine on a paper book that ran fast but the boy ran staff up in the . . . " Ms. Schneider, attempting to communicate with him, says: "You mean 'cut with a tork,' no, not a 'tork,' I mean a 'night' . . . no, a thing you cut food with!"

The two types of aphasia discussed and illustrated to this point are the more common syntactic and semantic aphasias. Other types occur. However, it is essential to know that there seldom is a "typical" patient. Communication-disordered brain-injured persons usually have a great variation and combination of communication problems.

The student might wish to explore in detail some of the very specific, perhaps less common language communication disorders stemming from brain injury. *Conduction aphasia*, in brief, deals with injury sustained in the pathways between language formulation and speech programming areas, leaving the patient with difficulties in forming syllables and words. *Transcortical sensory* and *motor aphasias*, rare and different from each other, are seen in patients with difficulties initiating speech or language. Other communication disorders one might investigate are *pure word deafness, aphemia, alexia (pure alexia)*, and *agraphia (pure agraphia)*. The Suggested Readings will guide you to supplementary and expanded details concerning these and other neurogenic language disorders.

CAUSES OF APHASIAS AND DYSARTHRIAS

A fairly common etiologic event is "*stroke*." This is a *cerebral vascular accident*, meaning that the blood supply to an area of the brain has been disrupted. Brain tissue can live for only a few minutes without a blood supply. When it dies, there is little expectation that it will heal or regenerate; the functions served by the involved neural tissue are lost. Other causes of brain injury include blows to the head as in automobile, vocational, or sports accidents or war-associated traumas. Tumor growth in the brain and other internal structural defects are also sources of aphasialike problems.

Damage in the posterior region of the cerebral cortex in the general area of the posterior temporal lobe may disturb language function. If the damage is more toward the front, a disorder of speech is more likely to result (see Fig. 5.2). Both types of damage are more likely to create communication disorders if they occur on the dominant side of the brain, or the left side in most persons, although right-sided brain injury can and does create communication problems in other dimensions such as inflection, rate, or stress patterns of speech.

Some of the dysarthrias stem from damage to brain centers deep within the brain. These are centers that check or regulate behaviors, and thus the speech function, being so very complex, can be disturbed by loss or damage. As each of the centers seems to have a unique role in motor behavior, the effect of damage to one center will probably be observed as different from damage to another center. Thus, the simple fact of "brain injury" gives no indication as to the nature of the communication disorder.

Attention should be placed upon other sources of language disorders associated with brain malfunctioning, whether due to known structural damage or not. Some of the degenerative processes that develop, often in older persons, may result in language disorders as well as other problems. *Senile dementia* (a group of aberrations of brain function), and *Alzheimer's* disease (perhaps one of the preceding) are but two of the brain disorders often associated with oral communication problems. The memory-based behavior disorders seen in some of these patients may include language difficulties. Psycholinguists, neuropsychologists, and language (speech) pathologists research these behaviors and defects not only to gain more detailed information on the disorders, but to better understand the functions of the brain in general. As the number of persons of older age increases, one might predict an increase in the number of such problems.

Neurogenic language disorders may be found in other populations, including children, but with uncertain prevalence. The effects of alcohol, drugs, and toxic wastes in water and air might be related to brain dysfunction and language disorders. Some of these have their effects prenatally, as for example, fetal alcohol syndrome. What may be important in such cases is the recognition of possible central nervous system involvement.

Peripheral nerve damage, such as a penetrating wound that severs a nerve to a muscle group, can occur almost anywhere in the body. As a nerve courses through other tissues (bone, fat, muscle), it is accessible to damage. Some of these damaged nerves can regenerate parts of their anatomy. Function can return, although not always to the preinjury level.

The injuries themselves and the damage they create are extremely variable. A penetrating wound may be caused by a bullet or a stabbing object. Injuries sustained in accidents may be penetrating or may move bones into damaging relationships to nerves serving the speech musculature. Surgeons must sometimes create (*iatrogenic*) nerve damage as they operate to remove life-endangering cancerous growths. Other tumors can encroach upon and interrupt the function of peripheral nerves to "speech organs." Obviously, the variety of causes for neurogenic disorders is great and as one might expect, management is equally variable.

EVALUATION

The assessment and management of neurogenic communication disorders in children and adults are best done by specialists knowledgeable in the areas affected by the neuropathology. The "team" members make their independent evaluations of the patient and then pool their information to better understand the full extent of the problems. They can then better develop recommendations and procedures in the treatment, or management, of the patient in his/her recovery.

Both children and adults may be evaluated in a similar manner, with the participating specialists varying. In the case of a child, one might expect a pediatrician to make an assessment. In both children and adults, an expert in neurology and its disorders plays an important role as a member of the team. Physical therapists participate in both the evaluation and the management phase. Occupational therapy contributes information on materials and procedures appropriate to the patient's problems and needs. A social worker can serve many functions in such a team: coordination of the team activities, communication of information pertaining to the patient, and counseling of the patient and family are among the several tasks performed by this specialist. And, of course, the speech-language pathologist plays an important role in both assessment and management aspects.

All team members utilize approaches that are as objective as their science permits. Standardized tests, instruments providing quantitative data, and careful collating of all forms of gathered information are among the ways in which an expert viewing a patient maintains objectivity. The speech-language pathologist has available well-known language batteries, aphasia tests. This specialist may utilize speech intelligibility tests that isolate aspects of speech; repeated muscle demands, such as sequenced tongue-lips-jaw movements in time segments, may clarify the basis for a dysarthric problem. The other team members may operate in a similar fashion from within their own disciplines.

Although we have emphasized the team approach—several specialists pooling information concerning a patient—there certainly are times when an expert functions alone. This is sometimes dictated by the nature of the employment: a geographic location where few other specialists work, a residential center for cerebral palsied persons, a pediatric clinic, a long-term care residential facility for the aged, etc. Some experts work in their own private clinics. Seeing communication-disordered patients without input from other disciplines may be a manner of working forced upon the clinician. However, written or other means of exchanging clinical information can often be developed for a particular patient's problems. An "ad hoc" team, lacking the face-to-face aspect, may not be ideal at all times, but is preferable to operating alone without the important information provided by other experts.

GENERAL MANAGEMENT APPROACHES

The treatment of neurogenic communication disorders varies from patient to patient. What was the nature of the injury, when did it occur (during or after the development of speech and language skills, for example), and what is the extent of the damage? The management is dependent upon the degree to which the effects of the injury are generalized throughout the body, how many other problems the individual has, and how important they are to everyday living and personal achievement. The treatment must also consider the communication modalities that may be affected by the brain injury: did it disturb speaking, writing, reading, listening, or some combination of these?

At the outset of the disorder, services to the patient are provided in the hospital when possible. The selected assessment procedures take place there, and variations of the tests may be repeated to determine the effects of treatment and of the passage of time. Whatever may be done to assist the patient to begin recovery of oral communication skills may take place in the hospital, as well as wherever the patient might go after hospitalization. Speech pathologists utilize a number of different approaches to assist the patient in recovery.

Biofeedback therapy is a means of teaching the patient to monitor his/her own speech activities and compare them with a standard. The approach may be auditory. A speech pathologist provides the model by saying a word or phrase, for example, and the patient is taught to compare his/her speech production with the model. Other senses are brought into the feedback training activities, also. The patient may need direction in placement of his/her articulators to produce certain speech sounds. Visual models may be presented, or tactile stimulation used as a guide. As biofeedback techniques grow in their sophistication and efficacy, they are likely to become more and more utilized in clinical management for aphasic patients.

Functional training involves the patient in more speech situations with modeling by the speech-language pathologist, a speech aide, or other person (e.g., the patient's wife or husband). Group therapy is another approach. Several persons with aphasia meet together under the direction of a speech pathologist. The activities include speech and language work; socialization and shared experiences take place to support and encourage the group members.

Some patients show little or no potential for oral speech because of their neurologic disorders. More and more nonvocal or augmentative communication techniques are developing for use with brain-injured persons and others. Instruments, computers, language boards, and other devices are becoming increasingly common for use with patients having neurogenic disorders. Some instruments have "joysticks" or wands that can be moved by little effort, such as a head turn or finger lift; these control a typewriter or other letter- or word-printing device. Computers and word processors are becoming most useful as augmentative communication devices. The older language boards, having words or pictures placed upon a board to which the patient points to communicate his/her wants, are still helpful in some instances. Future refinements in speech synthesizers that utter the words for the patient may well revolutionize augmentative communication instrumentation.

Treatment approaches are highly individualistic, especially formulated for each client. One point many clinicians use as a guiding principle is that brain tissue, once destroyed, does not regenerate. Thus the functions attributable to the affected area of the brain may be permanently lost. The outcome of this may be that the clinician will tell the patient that he/she may have to "live with" some part of the residual effects, or that another portion of the brain may be educated to compensate for the loss, or that the brain may be reprogrammed by therapeutic approaches to reorganize the lost or diminished skills.

Counseling of patients and those close to them is always an important part of the treatment program. Much advice must be given concerning the nature of the problem, its effects, and how to deal with the affected person in an understanding and perhaps helpful manner.

SUMMARY

Neurogenic communication disorders stem from abnormalities of the nervous system. They may occur as predominantly speech disorders. One may identify a deleterious effect upon breath support, phonation, resonance, or articulation, or some combination of these. The damage that creates such problems may occur in either the peripheral nerves serving the musculature or the central brain regions that exert overall control and coordination of the speech-producing system.

Neurogenic communication disorders also may be language disorders. One may identify a diminution of abilities in language reception or expression, or in a combination of these. The damage usually originates in brain centers and pathways, often from injury due to cerebral vascular accident, trauma, or degenerative brain disorders. The relative permanence of such damage is a significant aspect in understanding the communication disorder and the individual who exhibits it.

A third general area of neurogenic communication disorders is that associated with cognitive and memory problems. Some of these stem from disease or injury, while others may be tied to degenerative processes. Considerable research is providing a better understanding of the nature of the brain disorder and pointing to remediation approaches. Speech pathologists with high degrees of expertise now work with psycholinguists and neurology specialists (neurosurgeons, neuropsychiatrists, and others) to assist in the treatment programs for these patients.

Management or treatment of neurogenic communication disorders varies because of the great disparity in the nature of the original insult and the extent of its effects upon the individual. Compensatory skills, instruments, biofeedback, etc., become important, along with counseling of patients and their families. It may be a slow process, involving months of management and great understanding and empathy.

SUGGESTED READINGS

Several of the special anatomy textbooks for students of the speech and hearing sciences present chapters and illustrations limited to the neuroanatomy of speech and hearing. Much information about the entire nervous system and all body functions is not covered. The student will find more information concerning both the normal and the disordered nervous system in the following:

Kaplan, H. M. (1971). *Anatomy and Physiology of Speech,* 2nd ed. New York: McGraw-Hill.
Palmer, J. (1984). *Anatomy for Speech and Hearing,* 3rd ed. New York: Harper & Row.

Perkins, W. H., and R. D. Kent (1986). *Functional Anatomy of Speech, Language and Hearing.* San Diego: College Hill Press.

Zemlin, W. (1981). *Speech and Hearing Science: Anatomy and Physiology,* 2nd ed. Englewood Cliffs, NJ: Prentice Hall.

For more detailed and perhaps advanced information, the student should consult the chapters on neuroanatomy in any of the gross (visible with the naked eye) anatomy texts. For the following texts the most recent editions are given, but any earlier edition will suffice.

Anson, B. J. (Ed.) (1966). *Human Anatomy: A Complete Systematic Treatise,* 12th ed. New York: McGraw Hill. (Also known as *Morris' Human Anatomy.*)

Clemente, C. M. (1985). *Anatomy of the Human Body by Henry Gray,* 30th ed. Philadelphia: Lea & Febiger.

Romanes, G. J. (Ed.) (1981). *Cunningham's Textbook of Anatomy,* 12th ed. Oxford/New York: Oxford University Press.

For specialized neuroanatomy texts offering some detail, we recommend the following. Again, earlier editions are adequate.

Chusid, J. (1985). *Correlative Neuroanatomy and Functional Neurology,* 19th ed. Los Altos, CA: Lange Medical Publications. *The author puts a great deal of emphasis on function and provides clear explanations for much of it, especially reflexes and pathologies.*

Gardner, E. (1975). *Fundaments of Neurology,* 6th ed. Philadelphia: W. B. Saunders. *A text known for its straightforward, simplified explanations; it is popular in nursing and other medical professionals' education programs.*

Love, R. J., and W. G. Webb (1986). *Neurology for the Speech-Language Pathologist.* Stoneham, MA: Butterworth.

Study Questions

1. Explain how both a speech disorder and a language disorder could develop from the same injury to the brain.

2. Describe how you would identify the source of a speech problem as damage to a nerve outside the central nervous system. Would activities other than speech be involved?

3. In very general terms, explain how nerve impulses from the speech center in the cerebral cortex are modified by lower centers in the central nervous system. Consider the reverse situation, i.e., does Broca's area send impulses to the speech musculature without interruption?

4. Consider the relative locations of the speech and the language areas of the cerebral cortex; explain the difference in extensiveness of the resulting communication disorders resulting from damage to the front region and the back region of the cortex.

5. If the memory area of the brain becomes injured or imperfect in its functioning, what effect might this have on oral speech? Relate this question to the idea of "memory for words or language form" or other linguistic aspect.

6. Neurology includes sensation as well as neuromuscular activities. In a simple situation, explain how a dental anesthetic might create a speech problem. Then, take the "numbness" to a broader and more permanent problem, for example, complete numbness of the tongue. How might this affect speech production?

7. In some forms of cerebral palsy, voluntary control of the respiratory system is extremely difficult. For instance, a person with this problem might be exhaling under control (e.g., blowing out birthday candles) when the system automatically reverses itself to inhalation. How could this behavior create a speech problem?

8. Some degenerative forms of neuromotor diseases increase in severity through the day, as well as over weeks and months. A person with advanced myasthenia gravis might start the day with fairly adequate speech, including respiratory support, but experience increasing breakdown during the day. Discuss the effects on a person's daily living, beyond speech production, of such a problem.

9. Explain how an injury to the auditory areas of the brain can lie behind speech and language problems.

6

Stuttering

A cursory look at stuttering demonstrates its obvious character; its repetitions, pauses, and prolongations clearly interfere with the individual's plan to express thoughts orally. A smooth flow of speech cannot be produced; instead, disfluency occurs. The listener is usually struck with both the interruptions and the incompleted expression of an idea or thought. The stutterer himself/herself is held in check by what must seem to be an invisible, and apparently invincible, force. This speech disorder occurs more commonly in childhood and among boys. Its cause is uncertain, although there are a number of theories of etiology, which differ considerably. Such differences obviously lead to variable approaches in management.

Stuttering is an important if not common disorder. Its importance is largely due to the associated emotional component. This appears in the persons who listen to the stutterer, as they conjure up descriptive terms to describe the speaker beyond the speech interruptions, but more importantly it exists in the stutterer, with feelings of "fear and trepidation" arising in oral communication settings. The effects of these could certainly affect the growing child, and remediation becomes urgent.

INTRODUCTION

We emphasize here that stuttering is a speech disorder of considerable importance—not because it is so common but because it can be so debilitating. Various dictionaries indicate that "debilitate" means to weaken, to cause feebleness, to create a loss of strength. Stuttering can do just that. The thesis of this chapter is built around this point of view.

As a speech disorder, stuttering affects at the most about 1% of the total population. Some authorities suggest less, even as few as 0.5%. Others conclude that its prevalence may be diminishing. In considering its incidence—how often it occurs in a population—it is more than just interesting to note that males display stuttering more often than females. Prevalence studies show that between the ages of about three years and six years, the ratio may be nearly equal. Later, a ratio of about 4:1 develops suggesting either that more girls stop stuttering or that more boys begin to stutter.

113

Stuttering is commonly said to be a speech disorder of young children, but it can persist well beyond childhood years. It tends to diminish with maturity, with no commonly accepted reason provided for such a decrease. Of great importance is the age period between three and six years. It is during this time that stuttering is thought to commence. In fact, the age of three years may well be the time when the incidence peaks, when the majority of stutterers begin this manner of talking. Some children present evidence of stuttering with a rapid onset as young as two years of age. And, in some of these, the disorder may disappear just as suddenly.

When Mike rushed into the house calling out, "A kuh-kuh-cow jumped the fuh-fuh-fuh-fence!", most of the family became too busy to pay attention to his speech repetitions. Later in the day as he was describing the event to his father, he was more calm but equally repetitive: the kuh-kuh-kuh-cow and the fuh-fuh-fence, and even the guh-guh-grass and the tuh-tuh-tulips, gave evidence of his lack of fluency. Although Mike was only a little over 40 months old, his father said, "Tell me about it when you can talk better." One might conclude that the father's statement was not entirely supportive of Mike's speech effort, and could easily be interpreted by the boy as punishment.

Stuttering changes over the years in an individual. Different forms of stuttering behavior occur. A variety of accompanying behaviors and attitudes develop as the child grows and continues exhibiting this disorder.

As a preschooler, George was an active youngster attracting considerable attention, good and bad, from the adults in his home and elsewhere. His speech as it developed was clearly a kind of stuttering and was very demanding upon listeners who were trying to understand him. George would stutter and play and laugh and enjoy his world, at first. As time passed and he matured, George was made to recognize that his speech imposed and demanded. His effortful reactions to lessen his stuttering only seemed to increase the problem. In short, the more he tried the worse he became. Ultimately, in junior and senior high school George's speech was severely disordered. Worse, George knew he had such a problem and behaved accordingly. His social life was solitary. His interests and hobbies were activities that he could do alone. His school grades were average or below. Teachers did not call upon him and other students rarely just chatted with him. Others identified George, among themselves, as the "stutterer," and ultimately that was how George described himself.

DEFINITION/DESCRIPTION OF STUTTERING

A definition suggests that the object being defined is understood. Stuttering is not thoroughly understood, and thus there is some question about whether any definition would prove accurate. It seems wise to attempt a definition, but to quickly provide a description to forestall any permanent or hardened notion.

Stuttering is a disruption of the forward flow of speech. Most experts seem to accept this. It is an interruption in speech fluency. Stuttering can be extremely mild, with only minimal and perhaps unidentified speech flow disruption. This degree of interruption may be similar to that displayed by nearly every speaker at some time or other. A speaker can be "normally nonfluent" with a somewhat easy and perhaps relaxed way of repeating or pausing, without the tension that stutterers display. Examples are: the pause that occurs as one seeks the correct word, the hesitation to check that the listener is paying attention, the brief interruption to take a breath or to provide a moment of preparation for an important point, or the repeated word or phrase to provide emphasis or ensure clarity to an utterance. How does such normal nonfluency become stuttering? How does disordered fluency develop?

> When Roy talked about his favorite television cartoon (definitely not Porky Pig) he said, "I luh-luh-luh-like space cuh-cuh-cartoons." He had five repetitions in about one second; he was stuttering. Annie's statement on the same subject was, "Uh well, I guess, uh, I sorta like, uh, animal cartoons." She had three vocal pauses in a little over a second but they were more-or-less voluntary and she was not stuttering.

These behaviors are probably voluntary in the nonstuttering individual. The speaker chooses to use these devices for some communicative purpose. To be sure, this manner of speaking could become habitual. Yet, such a habit could be extinguished: since the speaker can "turn it on and off" with some degree of will, of volition, it is not a speech disorder in the narrowest sense.

The forward flow of speech can be impeded either by a cessation of talking such as an obvious hesitation, by repetition, or by prolongation of some aspect of speech. The stutterer may repeat a sound, a word, or a phrase a number of times in an utterance and apparently be unable to control this repetition. The repetition behavior is probably the first indicator of stuttering in the very young child. It can continue or may be replaced by some other interrupter.

It is very important, however, to note that all children (like all adults) may be disfluent on occasion. Repetitions can and do occur in what may prove to be a "normally disfluent" child. Disagreement exists among the experts as to the best method of distinguishing between what may prove to be a child who stutters and one who does not. Types and frequency of the disfluency receive the most attention in this process of distinguishing. One or two repetitions per utterance (a word or phrase) may be within normal limits, whereas five or more repetitions may indicate true stuttering, according to some specialists. Also, one may attempt to determine the degree of relaxed or tensed production in the disfluency.

> When little Jim first began to stutter, his speech was filled with repetitions. For example, if he wanted something to drink and his father asked him what he wanted, Jim might say: "Muh-muh-muh-muh-milk." Or, he might come rushing into the house to announce the presence of an animal visitor to the house with "Ki-ki-ki-kitty!" If the listener made some unpleasant comment about the way Jim talked, rather than the subject matter of his talking (i.e., the milk or the kitty), the boy may have felt that his speech was unacceptable, that the listener disapproved.

Stutterers show their speech problems in different ways. Professionals have called the specific difference the "block" or the "core behavior," or have used other labels. These indicate the instance of repetition, the specific sound prolongation, or the pause or hesitation. These signals can be accompanied by effort, by the speaker prolonging vocal sounds of various kinds. In addition, the stutterer might demonstrate the problem with gestures or facial grimaces accompanying the interrupted flow of speech. Combinations of these may occur in a single stutterer's collection of core behaviors that are called "stuttering."

Stutterers can often speak without stuttering, with no break in the flow of speech. These occasions are usually when there is some decrease in the level of the stutterer's responsibility to the listener, when there is less of a chance of reaction or punishment or even retaliation. Other stuttering-free occasions may take place when a stutterer is speaking with peers in choral fashion (as in repeating a poem, a pledge of allegiance, or a prayer as a group), when a stutterer speaks to an animal pet, or even when a stutterer sings or recites, and at other times when there is no outstanding possibility of unpleasant reaction to his/her speech. An explanation of these decreased stuttering events may focus on decreased speaker responsibility, or even change in physiologic (e.g., laryngeal) motor behavior.

As mentioned earlier, and as is the case in so many speech and hearing disorders, stuttering can vary in severity as well as in manner. A very mild stuttering problem may elicit only minimal reaction, by the speaker or by his/her associates. On the other hand, there are some persons whose speech is so severely disturbed that they are virtually "speechless." It might well be that persons at the latter end of the range of severity stutter for quite different reasons than do persons with only a mild degree of stuttering. In assessing the severity of stuttering, speech-language pathologists may count the number and types of interruptions in the speech of a stutterer, using these data not only to assess the severity but to establish objective bases for various comparisons (e.g., changes in the stutterer over time or differences among stutterers, etc.)

Two youngsters were referred to the speech pathologist because each was said to stutter. Anne would repeat the first syllable of a word on occasion, and at age five years, in kindergarten, it was thought that she should be more fluent. The speech clinician assessed the girl's speech in both structured and unstructured speaking situations. In both, Anne would repeat the initial syllable of a word once or twice, to be sure: "Th-th-thank you," or "Wh-where did I put my pencil?" Marty, on the other hand, required effort on the part of his listener to keep in mind his thought: "Wh-wh-what are we-we-we going to duh-duh-do?", "Sh-sh-shall I-I hang up muh-muh-my koh-koh-koah-coat?" Marty, at age six, is probably well into stuttering patterns as judged by the numbers of repetitions. Anne, on the other hand, could get by fairly well and with only an occasional repetition and might be called a "normally nonfluent" child.

WHAT CAUSES A PERSON TO STUTTER?

This section is identified by a question because it has not been easy to identify a single "cause of stuttering." Differences of opinion exist, and there are outspoken advocates of one or another etiologic condition or situation. Rather than be discouraged by the lack of a clear-cut causal factor, one might consider the possibility of there being several causes. What are some of the theories on the possible cause(s) of stuttering?

Breakdown Theories

Several opinions of stuttering causality involve a weakness or a breakdown in the physical or physiologic systems of the body responsible for smooth-flowing speech. The result is that the forward flow of speech is impeded. A number of concepts fall within this "breakdown" classification.

An early explanation was espoused by one of the first American speech pathologists, Lee Edward Travis. His idea, which caught the attention of many, including the non-speech specialists, is termed the cerebral dominance theory. The two hemispheres of the human brain behave somewhat differently from each other. The left hemisphere dominates in speech motor functioning. Because most of the anatomy of the speech system is approximately at the midline, one side of this neurologic system is the "leader." The cerebral dominance theorists suggest that in stutterers neither hemisphere of the brain takes the lead. The effect is that the muscles receive somewhat conflicting input, and the result is fragmented speech. The person develops unfortunate tactics, both physiologic and psychologic, to handle this neurologic conflict, and stuttering develops.

Another early speech pathologist, Jon Eisenson, also believed that the nervous system was the source of the stutterer's problem, but pointed to a slightly different aspect of the functioning. Although not an entirely close analogy, one might compare the events with the fault in a phonograph record that causes the needle to run in the same groove over and over again, repeating or perseverating the sounds recorded in that particular groove. In the human speaker, some sort of "short circuit" or other central nervous system aberration causes the stutterer to perseverate on a sound, syllable, or word. Perseveration is a general type of behavior disorder in which the person has a tendency to continue performing an act long beyond its appropriateness. A sort of reverberating cycle occurs during speaking.

There certainly seemed something wrong with Dara's mouth or with her tongue or throat when she talked because it took so much effort for her to say something. When her fourth grade teacher asked the class the name of the capital of Washington State, she volunteered to answer. Dara started with "Oh-oh-ohlym—" and her eyes closed tightly, her face turned red, and her hands grasped the desk edge as she leaned forward. And she slumped in defeat and dejection when the teacher interrupted: "Olympia! That's right, Dara."

These are but two "breakdown" theories. Although they were early notions of why people stutter, this does not mean that they are now extinct. Some aspects of each theory remain in other, more recent explanations.

Auditory Monitoring Theory

The variations of this approach are several, but essentially it suggests that stutterers hear themselves quite differently from how others, nonstutterers, hear themselves as they talk. Hearing oneself is auditory feedback. Generally, the child learns and the adult continues to use auditory feedback to check speech output against what he/she intended to say. The stutterer, according to this idea, has self-hearing that is out-of-phase or delayed from motor functioning. There is some conflict between input and output. This kind of conflict can result in hesitations, repetitions, or other stuttering-like behavior. Again, the additional actions and attitudes that the stutterer piles on to the speech problem make the stuttering grow and develop.

Psychoneurotic Theories

Because of his contributions to a better understanding of human emotions and behaviors, Sigmund Freud influenced the development of theories of stuttering causality. Specifically, the "repressed need" idea became the basis for this theory. This states that the stutterer has some unconscious need or drive that the conscious mind finds quite unacceptable to express out loud. How such a conflict may result in stuttering behavior is described in varying ways by clinicians who espouse the truth of the basic Freudian proposition. It is of interest to note that stuttering becomes a symptom of an underlying emotional problem. Such a problem may be demonstrated in other, perhaps unacceptable, behaviors. Treatment, then, would focus on the cause, not the symptom.

> Kenny had a short history of behavior problems in school and in his neighborhood. At school he was rough-playing around children younger than his 12 years, and had been heard to use some unacceptable language on the playground and in the bathroom. At home, Kenny had some toys and objects that belonged to neighborhood children, whose parents made objections and claims regarding their disappearance. When Kenny was referred to the school counselor, that specialist immediately heard what she thought was stuttering behavior in Kenny's speech. Long pauses, blinking of the eyes while effortfully giving his name, and repetitions—all were found in his repertoire. Since the initiating referral came about because of Kenny's behavior with other children, the counselor approached all of his problems, including the speech disorder, as an emotionally based disorder. She began a rather lengthy and in-depth study of Kenny's life, his family, and his various problems. Speech was considered a symptom of an underlying problem that gave rise to a number of unacceptable behaviors.

Learning Theories

More recent theories can be classified as learning-based: the stutterer has learned to stutter. The different approaches so classified, however, vary considerably in the mechanisms used. For example, one of the earliest of these theories was developed by Wendell Johnson, probably one of the most influential speech-language pathologists to examine stuttering. The term "diagnosogenic" has been applied because he believed that, in simplistic terms, the child stuttered because the parents (or others) placed that label on his/her speech behavior. Johnson and his followers have made a major point of identifying a child's normal speech as being occasionally nonfluent: normal nonfluency. But, for a potentially stuttering child, the parents bring unpleasant, perhaps punishing, attention to this otherwise normal behavior; they call the speech "stuttering" and the child a "stutterer." They clearly call the child's attention to unacceptable behavior. As a result, real and firmly established stuttering is what the youngster does to keep from stuttering, to avoid the punishment. The child learns to stutter. The focus here is on speech behavior resulting from punishing events.

> Mr. Frane probably loved his son Tom as much as any father. But when little Tom, at age five years, asked for some butter at the dinner table, and it came out "Ple-ple-please may I huh-huh-have some buh-butter?", Mr. Frane was irritated with the boy. His answer was: "No you cannot, until you quit that dumb stuttering and ask for it the right way. Now, slow down, think it out, and say it the way it should be said." Would that set up an easier, accepting environment for Tom's repeated request?

Another concept of the cause of stuttering is that held and taught by Joseph Sheehan: the "approach-avoidance conflict" theory. It emphasizes the child's learning to avoid speech troubles. Assuming that "trouble" (perhaps nonfluency in any situation) has occurred at one time and that the child remembers the event, he/she attempts to avoid that trouble when next encountering it. The child has problems in speaking and his/her way of avoiding those problems results in stuttering.

The field of stuttering has adopted some of B. F. Skinner's approach, often identified as "operant conditioning." How people learn behaviors, both acceptable and nonacceptable, can be related to a child who is learning to stutter. The child actually "operates" on his/her own speech by tensing, forcing, and ultimately by repeating or fixating. This might have come about because some other person or persons, e.g., the parents, called the child a stutterer in such a way that he/she found it unpleasant or punishing. Becoming frustrated by the failure to produce fluent speech, by the failure to control speech, the child's efforts (i.e., tensing, forcing, and repeating) caused him/her to learn to be a real stutterer. The implication may be that if the child operated on his/her speech to become a stutterer, then the child could operate on the stuttering to remove it.

Summary of Theories

The few theories presented here hardly begin to cover the many explanations for stuttering that have been offered. Today, outstanding scholars and clinicians are deeply involved in the task of better understanding the cause of stuttering and in developing the most productive means of treating the disorder. Many objections and rebuttals have been made to each of the theories presented. An acceptable "summary" is difficult to present, as well as to accept.

Apparently, speech does break down in stutterers, perhaps during times of tension or stress. It probably happens to some individuals more than to others, so that it occurs in people who will become stutterers more often than in people who will not become stutterers. Is there some physiologic weakness underlying the more frequent breakdown? If so, is it in the muscular system, or the neurologic system, or perhaps elsewhere in the body or mind of the speaker? It may well be that there are several causes of this speech disorder and that one of them (or some combination) may lead to stuttering.

THE PHASES OF STUTTERING

Some experts consider it important to identify various stages or phases through which a person passes in becoming a stutterer. This knowledge might ultimately lead to a better understanding of a possible cause of stuttering. It might also provide a point of entry into helping such a person when one has a better understanding of how far along the problem is, how developed the stuttering. However, although these are "stages" of development, there is no reason to believe that every potential stuttering person will pass through each stage in the same way, or will even pass through all stages. And most certainly not all potential stutterers will progress to true stutterers at the same rate.

Stuttering Acts

Many preschool children engage in some form of nonfluent speech behavior. The repetitions of initial sounds or syllables or words, or the hesitations or pauses, are probably the beginnings of the disorder. Most children do not have such seeds implanted in a fertile environment, and the stuttering problem never develops. But when it does, it may be convenient to assess the events that interrupt the forward flow of speech. Some call these events "core behaviors," others "blocks," while others simply note the stuttering events themselves.

When Morna reached four years of age, she was beginning to stutter without being very aware of it. Her parents didn't pay too much attention to her rather frequent repetitions of sounds and words, thinking she was a fast-moving, fast-thinking little girl. So when she said "Da-Daddy, there's a cuh-cuh-cat in the tuh-tuhree," they said nothing except, "Let's go see!"

Accessory Development

This may better be termed the "avoidance-escape-postponement" phase. Once the core behaviors have been established, it is not difficult for the incipient stutterer to add other behaviors or features. For example, the rate of repetitions, as well as signs of tension, might increase. A sort of "struggle behavior" may occur; the child forces and prolongs the speech act. This could continue through elementary school.

Morna's grandmother took care of her three days a week when Morna's parents worked. Grandma was more strict than the parents and had her opinions of what was correct and incorrect. Morna's speech repetitions were commented upon and Morna was strongly invited to "improve" her speech. As a result, the little girl tried to force out her words, if she could, or find another word for the word that had given her trouble earlier. Thus, she said "Guh-grandma, there's uhhhhh a . . . animal outside."

Avoidance Phase

Although stuttering is not really age-related, the stuttering child makes efforts to avoid it at some time—tries to release himself/herself, to escape from the clutches of whatever is causing the interruptions to speech flow. The development of external struggle that an observer can note are attempts to avoid or escape fluency failure. This youngster will avoid certain speech sounds, words, situations. The avoidance patterns may vary from time to time. At one point, the child might avoid all words beginning with an *s* because he/she had trouble with such a word last week. Next week a new speech sound can take its place.

Such children have strong aversions to special words that they have learned. There is no way stutterers can avoid a certain special set of words that make up their name, address, or school. They attempt to circumlocute, delay, or put off feared words. They select words other than feared ones. They learn to say, perhaps untruthfully, "I don't know" when asked a question by their teachers; this of course, can have an effect upon academic evaluations and progress. Others find that they have increasing speech difficulty with certain persons: their teachers, grandparents, a policeman, or others. This third phase of stuttering development, the avoidance phase, can have rather important effects upon the youngster's life in many ways.

> Sam is a 13-year-old who has stuttered for a number of years and still is unable to "control" his speech. He has developed avoidance behaviors around certain words, the most outstanding one being his own name. Sometimes, when a stranger asks his name, Sam will answer, "My parents' first child was Mary, and when I came along they had to find a boy's name, and they named me . . . well, they named me after . . . my name's . . . the same as . . . it's Sam!" Obviously, Sam goes to considerable lengths until he feels he can utter his own name. This avoidance, then circumlocution, is not uncommon; a stutterer might even go so far as to say, "I don't know" concerning something he/she knows quite well.

Associated Feelings Phase

A stutterer who makes it to this final developmental stage now has internal feelings about himself/herself tied in with stuttering. This is the most debilitating phase of stuttering. The association of fear, anxiety, or dread with speaking, and with stuttering, creates an important communication disorder. The child's great sensitivity and reactiveness to testing situations (and every time he/she speaks it is a testing situation) furthers the degree of disorder. A stutterer now identifies himself/herself as a stutterer—not a boy or girl, not a student, not an artist or whatever, but a stutterer.

> Half way through his ninth grade year, Herb was found to be a problem. Academically, his grades were far from satisfactory. Socially, he had few friends, sat in the rear of all his

classes, and rarely was seen talking with anyone. Teachers seldom called on him. He was "The Stutterer." If he was called on in class, Herb's initial reaction was surprise, then an effort to speak which resulted in a prolongation of "Uh," during which time a giggle or two could be heard in the classroom—and Herb would shrug his shoulders and gesture ignorance of the answer to the teacher's question. It was time-consuming, embarrassing, distracting, and often unprofitable to call on Herb in class. It did not happen often. What might people think of Herb's abilities?

Are there other phases? Perhaps there are. Probably the only one of some merit is that occurring as the child grows past puberty. It appears that between the ages of 16 and 20 years, some 80% seem to outgrow stuttering. This creates remedial as well as theoretic problems. Remedial problems occur because clinicians dare not wait to see whether a particular child will indeed outgrow the stuttering. Theoretic problems arise because outgrowing stuttering is a challenge to both the psychologic-based and the physiologic-based theories of causality. Specialists wonder what takes place in the person or in the environment that contributes to the decrease in stuttering. A theory of stuttering should accommodate such a change in speech fluency. However, knowing that about 80% of persons who stutter may outgrow the disorder in no way makes it less important as a disorder of childhood. In this period of growth and development, the dynamics of the child's relationships and behaviors are laid down for the future, and stuttering may have its effects on that future.

EVALUATION

Before any remediation approaches may be tried, the speech-language pathologist makes a careful evaluation. Its nature is heavily dependent, as one might expect, upon the age of the stutterer, the stage of development of the stutter, the effects on the child and others, and so on. Of course, any evaluation is based upon a careful case history, detailing health, social, personal, and other problems that might be related, as well as a history of the stuttering, searching for the beginnings and development of the problem.

A questionnaire for the parents, or for the stutterer, is often helpful. Here, not only is the stuttering itself investigated but the clinician seeks for reactions and attitudes as well as effects of the communication disorder. The speech-language pathologist questions personal habits, social activities, school work, and other areas of behavior that might be affected by the stuttering.

And, of course, measures of the stuttering are made. The type of stuttering, its severity and duration, and the reaction of the stutterer to his/her own speech difficulty are among the aspects studied by the clinician. It is necessary to listen and watch as the stutterer speaks. Even the nature of the speaking situation is important; should the evaluation consist of only the speech-language pathologist and the child? Should the clinician observe interpersonal relationships and speech activities in other situations, such as between parent and child, between another child and the stutterer, and so on? The clinician knows that there are differences in speaking abilities from one environment to another, and this is also true for stutterers. There are differences in stuttering behavior between children and adults, between incipient stuttering and fully developed stuttering, among other differences that occur.

From these and other evaluative procedures, the speech-language pathologist develops an impression of the nature of the problem, the nature of the stutterer, and perhaps a tentative plan of management for remediating the communication disorder.

GENERAL MANAGEMENT APPROACHES

From the description of stuttering given in this chapter, it should be easy to conclude that the therapy depends greatly upon the stutterer. One would hardly expect the same understanding or the same behaviors from a very young stutterer as from an adult stutterer. Another reason for the variability in approaches is the difference among clinicians' opinions as to what stuttering is and what causes it. The approach used by a clinician who subscribes to a breakdown theory will certainly differ from that of a clinician grounded in a psychoneurotic-based theory. So, in general, there is some variation among professionals in the way they try to help stutterers. However, some general activities and approaches can be described that should not offend any theorist or clinician.

Identification

A very early aspect of the remediation program for stutterers is a careful study of the stutterer and the stuttering. The results of this study are importantly related to the kinds of goals that the clinician establishes for the client and the kinds of techniques selected to reach those goals. Illustrative of this would be the clinician's task of studying the individual stutterer. Who is this person?

> A boy of ten years who is said to stutter is interviewed thoroughly. It is important to determine whether this child feels himself to be a stutterer. If he does, is this a serious source of concern for the child? Attention may be placed on the child and his speech. If he does not, then a different approach might be utilized. Who *is* the concerned person: a parent, a teacher? And who needs the remediation? An adult man who is a stutterer needs an equally thorough evaluation to examine the relationship between the speech disorder and his self-expectations, goals, and general social behavior. Does he have generally lowered self-expectations because of his fluency failures? Are his personal goals limited by his stuttering? Is he not as social an individual as another person who is similar to him but does not stutter?

As noted earlier, the initial evaluation and subsequent management are not simple procedures. They require skill in interviewing and patience in awaiting responses. The responses can be difficult to observe; one tends to participate in the struggle a stutterer demonstrates. The information being sought is important in order to describe the client in every way possible. The more information the clinician has about the client and the problem, the more valid is the ultimate remediation program. Therapy (or remediation) is nothing more than continuous reevaluation, constantly evaluating the client and the disorder as changes occur during the therapeutic process.

The Child Stutterer

With a child who stutters, one thing often done by the speech clinician is to determine just when this behavior first occurred. Who is involved? Who labels the child's talking as "stuttering?" What is going on in the child's environment at that time? Are these factors important in management?

The situations in which the child's stuttering are noticed must be understood. If there is some sort of pressure on the child in those circumstances, it is wise to lessen that pressure. The demand to speak and to speak "correctly" could be determined, and if present, decreased in its intensity. A permissive speaking environment could be sought and encouraged. And removal of any reactions suggesting punishment or rejection should certainly be accomplished. If possible, prevention of stuttering or the further development of stuttering is an important target for the speech-language pathologist.

For the child who stutters, a major aspect of the remediation is performed through the parents, teachers, or other important persons in the child's life. The child himself/herself can be offered therapeutic situations to develop the permissive and demand-free speech activities that can be so productive. Depending upon the child's own attitudes, openings can be developed for discussing the problem and its effects.

The Older Stutterer

The clinician's rationale for stuttering remediation is dependent upon his/her education, experience, and what he/she identifies as the nature of the client's stuttering. There is no single universal therapeutic approach to stuttering, although various methods involving learning theory seem to be popular and effective.

An early stage of therapy involves self-evaluation of the problem by the stutterer. What does he/she do when stuttering? What sort of speech changes occur? What associated and accompanying physical and emotional changes can be noted? Are these things an important part of the stutterer's underlying behavior, or are they some things the stutterer does as part of the stuttering? Looking at these is the beginning of objectifying them. The stutterer isolates each—for example, the unhelpful eye blinks and head jerks, the tension and worry that interfere with oral communication. Can they be eliminated to better the situation? Decreasing these behaviors is an important step to decreasing the apparent severity of the stuttering. Even working toward "normal disfluency" can be an important target.

The work to objectify the stuttering and its accompanying associated characteristics starts to remove the stutterer's sensitivity toward the speech disorder. In the process of learning that these things are events with causes and effects, the stutterer learns to desensitize himself/herself to them. Although not really "accepting" the stuttering, he/she has placed it into some real perspective to examine. This takes it from the realm of mystery, fear, and other emotional reactions. It gives the stutterer "something to work on."

The speech clinician, though continuing to explore the problem with the stutterer in the process of desensitization, leads the client into activities designed to better control speaking abilities. A multitude of tactics is possible. Developing easy, relaxed breath control during speaking demonstrates to the stutterer that those unusual behaviors tied in with breathing are not necessary: the shallow breathing or the gasping inhalation. Another activity is to engage in prolonged speech movements with easy phonation. Removing the forcefulness that stutterers may incorporate in speaking further illustrates that they have control. It also may demonstrate that they can speak without severe stuttering. An approach that utilizes a specific "method" in this vein is the "fluency shaping" technique in which the stutterer moves from one aspect of speaking to another, under the modeling established by the clinician.

> Bobby's speech pathologist was able to make the clinical setting comfortable. Being in the room became more pleasant than unpleasant. The speech pathologist was clearly accepting, not punishing. After a few sessions, Bobby was asked to use his speech mechanism easily and without force; he found he could hum easily. He next found that he could initiate humming, and in the same breath move easily to a vowel production. Bobby then discovered a few words that seemed close to that activity, such as "ma" or "me" or "moo." Deliberately slow, easy, prolonged speech activities graduated to more and more complex utterances. With ample rewards from his speech pathologist, Bobby moved closer and closer to more controlled and noninterrupted speech, although it took weeks for each little step.

Such activities can be programmed. The stutterer commences work at a certain basic stage, then works through progressive step-by-step advancement phases. Depending upon the history of the stutterer, it can be a time-consuming procedure. Some stutterers have talked this way for some years. Their neuromotor systems may be programmed for them to stutter. Their emotional systems may be built around the stuttering. Their social life—family and friends and events—may be structured around stuttering. So, although it may not be difficult to demonstrate simple speech improvement in a therapy room, a different and time-consuming effort may be needed to carry improved speech patterns to outside-of-therapy situations.

The internal feelings, the most severe problem with which advanced stutterers must deal, must be resolved. Progress can be determined by these feelings, and if progress does occur, regression can be tied in with these deep-seated emotional behaviors. Whatever the approach, stutterers of advanced age need to have some grasp of the nature of their stuttering and their own feelings about the speech problem. With increased understanding of both aspects, less effort may be necessary in the speech act. With decreased struggle and some positive steps suggested by the clinician, stuttering behavior can decrease in frequency and severity.

It should be evident from these few paragraphs that approaches to stuttering differ from clinician to clinician and from case to case. More importantly, there is probably no single program that is universally applicable to relief of this disorder. Each clinician must develop his/her own approach, unique to a particular client, depending upon the nature, degree, history, and characteristics of the stuttering behavior. In this way, stuttering therapy parallels remediation approaches in many of the other speech disorders.

SUMMARY

Stuttering is an interruption in the forward flow of speech. Stuttering behaviors are hesitations, repetitions, prolongations, and circumlocution. These may be accompanied by various other behaviors, e.g., postural changes, facial grimaces, and inappropriate vocalizations. Any of these cause the speech to be identified as disordered, for any can draw negative attention to the process of speaking, decrease speech intelligibility, or cause the speaker (stutterer) to have feelings of lessened self-worth.

The problem most frequently develops early in childhood and continues well through the school-age years. The core behaviors may occur in the speech of a child who is developing normally and who may never become a stutterer; or, to put it another way, a child whose speech has interruptions may be essentially normal, having "normal nonfluent" speech. Why these interruptions in the forward flow of speech become true stuttering is the object of much study and some disagreement. The theories range from physiologic weaknesses and breakdown, to emotional or personality bases, to learned behaviors. The possibility of multiple causal factors must also be considered. Whatever the cause, the stuttering child may develop through phases from easy repetitions to severe, nearly speechless behaviors with associated emotional problems. It should be apparent that stuttering might interfere with many aspects of the child's life: family, social, and academic.

Remediation approaches vary along with the etiologic theories. The management technique matches the causal factor that the clinician believes to be in effect. If it is considered a physiologic breakdown, a physiologic approach might be utilized; if it is thought to be an emotionally based problem, counseling would be considered; in the case of the learned theory possibility, a learning approach might be used. In each case, there are many reports of successes and some failures. What is surprising is that stuttering is often "outgrown." There are few geriatric stutterers.

The research needs in this disorder are several. The mechanisms involved in the "outgrowing" process are under study. Other investigators are looking at the causal factors and others at the remediation approaches. Obviously, stuttering is a complex disorder and it is far from solved. Yet there are many fine speech pathologists successfully assisting persons who stutter to communicate better.

SUGGESTED READINGS

Bloodstein, O. (1987). *A Handbook on Stuttering,* 3rd ed., Chicago: National Easter Seal Society for Crippled Children and Adults. *A readable discussion of the disorder by an eminent authority in the field, available through a local Easter Seal Society.*

Curlee, R. F., and W. H. Perkins (Eds.) (1984). *Nature and Treatment of Stuttering: New Directions.* San Diego: College Hill Press. *Edited by two authorities on stuttering, this compendium presents objective information using a sensitive approach in tone and content. It includes a very interesting chapter by Costello and Ingham on viewing stuttering as an operant disorder.*

Van Riper, (1973). *The Treatment of Stuttering.* Englewood Cliffs, NJ: Prentice-Hall. *An extremely thorough review of the varying approaches to remediation of the stuttering disorder. A standard reference for speech pathologists, requiring some background (at least Van Riper's* Nature of Stuttering) *for ease of understanding.*

Van Riper, C. (1982). *The Nature of Stuttering,* 2nd ed. Englewood Cliffs, NJ: Prentice-Hall. *This became the most authoritative textbook source for information about the disorder. It carefully discusses definition, development, phenomenology, and theories of causality, and provides a careful synthesis. This book does no more than hint at the treatment of stuttering; the author delves into this topic in another text.*

Van Riper, C. (1984). Stuttering. Chapter 8 in *Speech Correction: Principles and Practices,* 7th ed., pp. 257–336. Englewood Cliffs, NJ: Prentice-Hall. *One of the most sensitive of the writings about stuttering, from a foremost expert in the field. He approaches the objective as well as the more emotional aspects of the disorder from the perspective of years of experience in working with persons who stutter. The chapter is replete with clinical illustrations and should give the reader a clear understanding of the nature and effects of the disorder.*

Wingate, M. E. (1976). *Stuttering Theory and Treatment.* New York: Irvington. *A scholarly analysis of theories of causality and approaches to treatment of stuttering, research-based and objectively presented. A stimulating contribution from an authority in the field.*

Study Questions

1. Clarify for yourself what "normal nonfluency" is by listening to average people talking at coffee breaks or parties or elsewhere (do not analyze radio or television dramatic or news programs in which the speakers follow printed scripts). Note the variation in pausing, the hesitations, the repetitions of sounds and words. Is common, everyday, social speech fluent without interruption?

2. Test the emotional impact of stuttering yourself. Go to the bookstore and ask for one of the texts in the Suggested Readings list. But do so by imitating stuttering. Repeat three or more times, not less, the initial sounds in the names of the text. Look in the eyes of the clerk as you say it. Note your feelings as well as the reaction of the clerk. Does he/she look away? Attempt to help you? Walk out? Make a comment about your speech?

3. Ask those you know what they believe to be true of stuttering. What do they think it is? Do they have opinions as to what causes it? Do they think a stutterer is different, in some way, from nonstutterers? What effect would people with such opinions have on a stutterer when they actually meet one?

4. Read some of the research literature on stuttering. Look up the authors in the Suggested Readings list in professional journals such as *Journal of Speech and Hearing Research* or *Journal of Speech and Hearing Disorders* available in your university library and read some of their articles. Find an article about stuttering in a "lay" magazine and compare it with the journal articles.

7

Speech Disorders Caused by Anatomic Defects

In this chapter we present a few of the anatomic defects that can lead to communication disorders. If you do not have an extensive background in human anatomy, you may need to refer to appropriate diagrams or even to other texts in anatomy and physiology. Many new terms may appear in this chapter; see the Glossary.

Remember that this is a "survey" book. Each anatomic area and each physiologic activity will demand more attention than is given here. Keep in mind that "anatomy" (and "anatomic") usually refers to the form, the structure; for example, the tongue, the vocal folds, and the lungs. "Physiology" (and "physiologic") commonly suggests actions, behaviors, or movements; illustrative of this are swallowing, breathing, and phonation.

We discuss here all the basic, normal anatophysiologic aspects, some examples of defects, their effects on oral communication, and some remediation approaches. The disorders discussed are probably the most common; however, there are many variations in the causes, effects, and management.

INTRODUCTION

Speech-language pathologists and audiologists may serve persons with defects of the vocal tract, the nervous system, and other anatomic regions associated with the communication process. Some of these disorders of structure and function stem from *prenatal influences,* others from growth and development failures, and still others from *injury, neoplasms, or surgery.* These problems may not even be directly associated with oral communication. The rather intensive study and observation required of students in this specialty provide a background that often can be applied to clinical management procedures for anatomic or physiologic disorders even when there is no speech problem.

129

This chapter concerns anatomic and physiologic abnormalities. *The actual speech problems that might be associated with structural deformities—articulation, phonation, resonance, and language—have been discussed in earlier chapters.* When reference is made here to one of these areas, the reader is urged to review the appropriate chapter.

Although speech and language disorders occur in the defects discussed in this chapter, often it is the anatomic and physiologic problems that become the focus of attention. In such cases, the speech-language pathologist usually serves as a member of a multidisciplinary team. The members of the team are involved because of their special skills in treating the patient's problems. Laryngologists, plastic surgeons, prosthodontists, psychiatrists, social workers (and other counselors), and neurologists are among the specialists who frequently serve patients, in addition to the communication specialist.

> A recent team panel (or staffing) for a youngster with a repaired cleft palate included two speech pathologists, four plastic surgeons, an audiologist, an orthodontist, a prosthodontist, an otolaryngologist, a geneticist, four public health nurses, and a coordinator. The patient was a 14-year-old boy who had some mild residual hypernasality and articulation problems, a hole in the posterior palatal region, teeth that were in poor condition and in malocclusion, earaches and some hearing loss, and a history of failing to appear at specialty appointments. After considerable discussion and a careful "look" at the boy, it was agreed that he should receive intensive trial speech work, immediate dental care including orthodontic treatment, closure of the hole (*fistula*) by either plastic surgery or prosthesis, and recall to the panel in six months. The public health nurse assigned to the child's case was to ensure that he kept appointments and to coordinate treatments among the specialists.

The patient's problems and needs dictate the nature of the specialty team. At times, it is the speech-language pathologist who provides primary care. At other times, another specialist must first be involved, and then the patient may be referred back to the communication specialist for later follow-up. It is decidedly dependent upon the patient's problems and needs, and upon the nature of the anatomic or physiologic disorder itself and the ways in which it differs from the normal structure and function. A review of "normal aspects" is in order before one can establish what abnormal or disordered structure and function may be.

REVIEW OF PERTINENT ANATOPHYSIOLOGIC AREAS

It would be helpful at this point to review the anatomy and physiology of the vocal tract areas by referring to earlier chapters. More in-depth information from sources specifically focused upon these areas (see Suggested Readings) will provide a broader knowledge base.

In the structural review, it is important to keep in mind both biologic and speech functions; each is obviously important to the client. At times the speech pathologist is more interested in one than the other. Knowledge of both may provide the necessary skill to serve disorders of the biologic or the speech disorder, or both. As you read the spatial and structural descriptions that follow, remember that herein lie the bases of malformation or malfunction. Nearly every anatomic entity noted here may be involved in some disorder of mastication, swallowing, or speech. There is ample reason for the speech pathologist to have detailed knowledge of these aspects of the vocal tract.

The vocal tract commences in the larynx at the vocal folds and is related to vocalization in general (hence "vocal"), and it is a series of related chambers (hence "tract") through which pass air and sound for speech production. These chambers are formed by anatomic structures—walls and boundaries that partially encase the chambers. Movement of these walls is usually possible. Such structures and movements contribute to the production of acoustic events that form speech. The anatomic areas discussed here are illustrated in Figures 7.1 and 3.1; some points appear in one and not in the other. We also refer you to any standard anatomy or physiology text, some of which are noted in the Suggested Readings.

Some of the life-supporting anatomy that is shared in oral communication will not be covered in detail. The lower respiratory tract—the trachea, bronchi, and lungs—provides the energizing force for speech production. Some of the anatomic and physiologic sources of speech disorders are found in this sub-vocal tract region. As described in earlier chapters, equally important to speech production are the controlling, coordinating, and initiating roles of the nervous system. Again, disorders of speech and language may stem from structural anomalies therein. Lastly, a critical factor in oral communication is played by the auditory system; this will be discussed in Chapter 8. It is important to survey the embryonic (prenatal) and postnatal development of the vocal tract.

DEVELOPMENT OF THE VOCAL TRACT

Survey of Embryonic Development

In the first few days after fertilization, the embryo becomes elongated and a head-end and a tail-end appear. In the section that will become the surface of the face, the eyes are situated wide apart. The ears form from a low position but ultimately migrate to higher locales in the head-end. The nasal openings share an opening with the mouth. Projections grow from the sides, toward the front, ultimately fusing with middle structures. The fusion, toward the end of the second month of embryonic development, forms the completed nose and upper lip. This usually occurs at the end of the embryonic period and the beginning of the fetal period.

Internally, the palate arises as two separated shelves from the sides of the combined nasal and oral chambers. The space between the shelves in the embryonic period is occupied by the tongue. As the lower jaw bone, the mandible, forms and develops downward, it lowers the tongue. This allows the two palatal shelves to meet and fuse in the midline, thus forming the palate, the separation between the nasal and oral spaces. This is completed by the end of the third month of development.

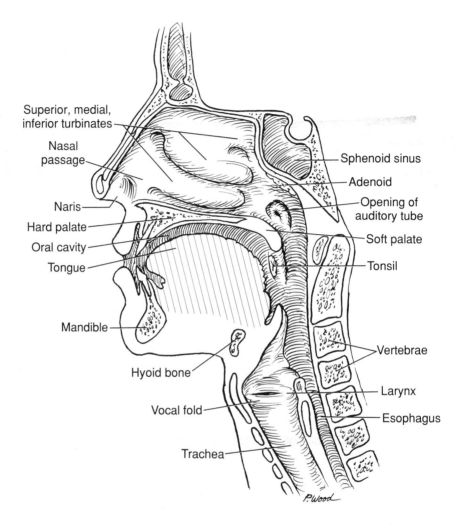

Figure 7.1. The Vocal Tract

During the first few weeks of intrauterine life, the palate of the developing embryo stopped in its progress toward fusion. So, at the time of her birth, Heidi was found to have a cleft palate. The reasons for this fusion failure never became completely clear. A plastic surgeon was consulted by Heidi's pediatrician. The latter was involved because of the infant's problems in feeding: food would enter her mouth and often pass out through her nose rather than down the digestive tract. Special feeding approaches were necessary to maintain her health. Knowing that children with palate clefts often develop hearing problems because of failure to ventilate the middle ear through the auditory tube, the plastic surgeon also called upon an otolaryngologist to examine Heidi. When she was about 18 months old, Heidi's palate was closed surgically by the plastic surgeon. Her feeding became more regular. She also greatly increased her potential for good speech, a status that was followed over the next several years by regular visits to a speech pathologist.

Postnatal Development

The soft palate is seemingly very long, suspended down behind the tongue, even overlapping the upward-thrusting epiglottis. In the newborn infant, this approximation of the two structures assists the child in swallowing and breathing at the same time, such as during suckling. This ability to carry on the two activities concurrently is lost as the child develops. A vertical increase in head size, and thus in the pharyngeal regions, separates the velum from the epiglottis, and the concurrent breathing-swallowing ability disappears.

As the child develops further, the vertical growth of the head provides increased volume in the nasal chambers. The nasopharynx increases in vertical dimension, as do the other pharyngeal divisions. The larynx, and especially the hyoid bone, seem to lower in the head-neck region.

In the first year of life, the brain continues to grow, expanding not only in size (thanks to the cartilaginous *fontanelles* of the skull that provide for growth) but in nervous tissue structure and complexity. As the nervous system's anatomy develops, so does the potential for increased complexity of function, including speech.

Through the childhood years, a large number of growth changes occur, some of which are important to speech. More bone tissue develops. Lymphoid tissues found in the pharyngeal region (*palatine tonsils, pharyngeal tonsils,* and *lingual tonsils*) grow, then usually diminish as puberty approaches. The *mandible* continues to grow; the chin is formed. The *ramus* of the mandible changes angles from oblique to more acute. The larynx begins to enlarge at about the time of puberty. This enlargement is especially noticeable in the male. The vocal folds within also grow, causing a lowering of the fundamental frequency in the voice of the male by nearly an octave, and in the female perhaps by only a couple of semitones. Before this, the male and female larynges are extremely similar, and few differences are observable between children's voices whether male or female.

Neuromuscular skills increase throughout the growth period. Changes in hormonal balances occur. Muscular development takes place, due to activity in the growth centers of the bones. Bone growth and bone fusion continue into the third decade of life, if not beyond. Throughout life, as one ages, body changes continue.

REVIEW OF THE VOCAL TRACT

Recall that the *vocal folds* are found within the larynx. Their biologic purpose is to act as a valve against the entrance of foreign objects (e.g., crumbs, drops of saliva) into the lower airway and lungs. The speech purpose of the vocal folds is to come together into the exhaled airstream to vibrate and produce phonation.

Air and phonation enter the pharynx from the airway below. The air and sound enter the lowest portion of the pharynx, the *laryngopharynx* (or *hypopharynx*). The lower pharynx contributes to resonance of the voice and serves as the tube carrying food into the lower digestive tract. Examine the figures illustrating the relationships among the larynx, laryngopharynx, and the esophagus (see Figs. 3.1, 4.4, 7.1). Note the routes taken by air in respiration and by food in *deglutition* (swallowing) (Figs. 7.2, 7.3).

Following his head injury that resulted in a complex of neurologic disorders, Sam McCardle showed serious problems in eating and swallowing. In fact, some portions of food and drink were *aspirated* into the trachea and perhaps lungs, providing a potential for dangerous aspiration pneumonia. Among his related problems were speech disorders, largely dysarthric, as well as palatal paralysis. Careful radiographic evaluation of Sam's swallowing pattern with small bits of barium-coated food showed that the larynx did not elevate nor did the *cricopharyngeal sphincter* release to receive the bolus of food. Thus, any food descending to that region could be passed into the airway, until the sphincter finally allowed food to enter. The speech pathologist making the evaluation determined that there were some special reflex-training techniques that might be applied to ameliorate the problems.

The lower pharynx continues upward to become the middle pharyngeal chamber, the *oropharynx*. This space serves both the digestive and respiratory systems, as

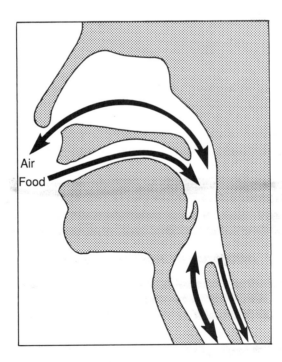

Figure 7.2.   Upper Vocal Tract: Breathing and Eating

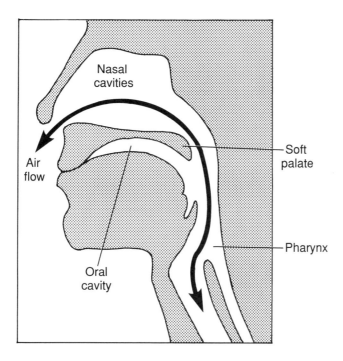

Figure 7.3. Breathing: Normal Nasal Air Flow

well as vocal resonance. Food from the oral cavity (Fig. 7.4) enters and is moved downward into the laryngopharynx and ultimately the esophagus. The respiratory function is served as inhaled air from the nose and mouth and exhaled air from the larynx and trachea traverse the chamber. The oropharynx continues upward, via the *velopharyngeal port,* to join with the *nasopharynx.* The function of the oropharynx in speech is to join with other chambers in air transport for oral speech production and to carry sound for resonance and voiced phoneme articulation.

The third pharyngeal division, the *nasopharynx,* serves only the respiratory function biologically. It does serve speech in English by adding a nasal resonance quality to the voice in forming the nasal consonants. It can be separated from the oral pharynx by the combined actions of the soft palate (*velum*) and the muscular pharyngeal walls in *velopharyngeal closure* (discussed in "The Oral Cavity"). This separation is an essential activity in swallowing and in the production of most English speech sounds. The patent (open) velopharyngeal port provides nasal coupling with the oral pharynx in vital breathing and in the production of the nasal consonants. Examine Figures 7.2 and 7.3 illustrating the way in which the nasal airway chambers are coupled with the pharyngeal chambers in breathing.

The anterior communication of the nasopharynx is with the two nasal passages. Perhaps the most important anatomic features of the nasopharynx are the two open-

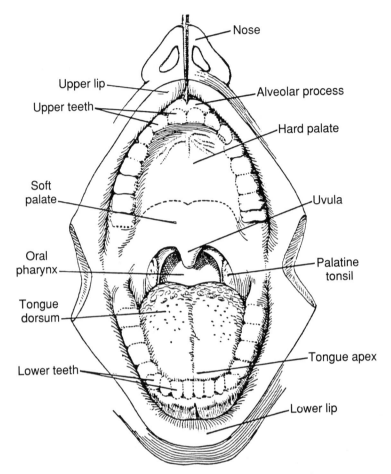

Adapted from clinical forms used at Memorial Hospital, New York.

Figure 7.4. The Oral Cavity

ings into the canals to the middle ears. Each opening is into the *auditory* (Eustachian) *tube.* Its function is to provide drainage of the middle ear when mucus or other fluids form, as well as to provide ventilation. The cartilage of the tube usually is collapsed, and thus the tube is usually closed. It is opened, when necessary, by one or perhaps two important muscles. This occurs during swallowing, yawning, and when the person moves from one air pressure environment to another, such as in driving over a mountain pass, moving rapidly in an elevator, or changing altitude in an airplane.

Jennie is a three-year-old with a history of earaches and running ears, sore throats, mouth breathing, and more recently an important hearing impairment. Her otolaryngologist, to whom she was referred by the audiologist (who discovered the hearing impairment), found that she had large adenoids that blocked off the auditory tubes. With fluid build-up in the middle ear and with possible infections, the middle ear health was less than desirable. The otolaryngologist inserted ventilation tubes through her tympanic membranes, which provided for ventilation of the middle ear and some drainage of *fluids,* and also prescribed appropriate medications for the infections. After a period of several months, repeat examination by the physician demonstrated a healthy ear, and the audiologist also found significantly improved hearing. Jennie will be carefully followed annually, if not more frequently, to ensure that repeat infections, and thus hearing impairment, do not occur.

The mouth, more properly termed the *oral cavity,* is the site of major speech activities. Visible through the mouth opening is the tongue. Its large upper surface (the *dorsum*) is horizontally oriented (Fig. 7.4). This and other tissues of the region serve the biologic functions of taste and touch. The tongue is an elegantly flexible and maneuverable device, important to chewing, swallowing, and speech.

The tongue is not "the" organ of speech, but it is certainly an extremely important structure, not only for speech but for other life-supporting functions. The tongue maintains food between the surfaces of the opposing teeth during chewing. If it did not do this, the pieces of food might fall off the teeth and not be pulverized in the *mastication* process.

The tongue is very important for another function of life support: *deglutition* (swallowing), necessary for the transport of the masticated food *bolus* through the oral cavity. The bolus is chewed food partially dissolved by saliva and coated by mucus in the mouth. Normal swallowing of this bolus is a four-stage procedure.

1. *Preparatory stage:* The food that has been chewed is placed upon the dorsum of the tongue, the lips are closed to prevent the escape of any part of the bolus, and the upper and lower teeth are approximated.

2. *Oral stage:* With the food on its dorsum anteriorly, the tongue tip is elevated to the alveolar ridge or anterior bony palatal region. The remainder of the tongue dorsum is elevated sequentially from front to back against the palate. The bolus is forced by the moving contact region toward the back of the mouth and through the faucial isthmus into the pharynx. This takes about one second. Velopharyngeal closure (Fig. 7.5) prevents arriving food from entering the nasopharynx or the nasal passages.

3. *Pharyngeal stage:* The food has now been thrust rapidly into this muscular tube—the pharynx—which has been occluded (by velopharyngeal closure) at its upper end. A sphincterlike action is repeated as the pharyngeal wall muscles contract sequentially from top to bottom to force the bolus downward *(peristalsis).* As the bolus passes downward from the oral pharynx, the opening to the larynx is closed and the food slides into the laryngopharynx. The esophagus opens to receive the food, then closes behind it as it passes down through the digestive tract. Passage through the oral cavity and pharynx should take no more than ten seconds, probably less, before the bolus enters the esophagus.

4. *Esophageal stage:* The bolus has entered the muscular esophagus. The walls

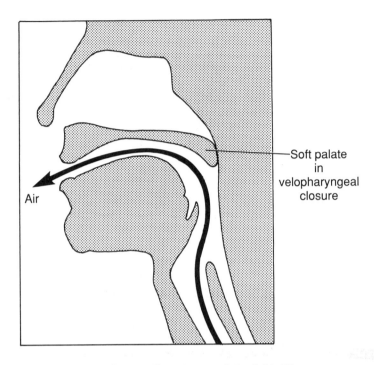

Figure 7.5.   Talking: Normal Oral Air Flow

of this tubular system continue the peristaltic action to pass the food downward toward the stomach.

> Mabel Ferdinand was found to have a cancerous growth beneath her tongue. It was essential that it be removed. The surgery required was also forced to interrupt cranial nerve XII (hypoglossal nerve) that serves the muscles of the tongue. This paralyzed the tongue. Among the various problems resulting (including numerous speech distortions) were in chewing and swallowing. Mabel's speech pathologist took her to a nearby prosthodontist who had experience with patients of this type. Together, the two specialists examined, fabricated, and fitted a plastic prosthesis for the roof of Mabel's mouth. This occupied oral cavity space. Since the tongue muscles could move only minimally during chewing and swallowing, the prosthesis made the distance the tongue had to move considerably less. It facilitated the two important biologic functions, and increased Mabel's potential for speech improvement.

THE ORAL CAVITY

It is important to remember that the structures in the mouth that serve chewing and swallowing also serve speech production. The tongue (Fig. 7.4) is important to the production of vowel sounds, as it changes its position in the oral cavity to vary resonance conditions. Such terms as "high vowel" and "back vowel" generally refer to tongue positions required to produce certain vowel sounds. In consonant production, too, the tongue plays a prominent role. In forming constrictions of the vocal tract at certain locales, it contributes to oral formations that affect air flow and pressure.

Muscular activities to groove the tongue, to elevate its apex, to raise its posterior dorsum, or to retract the pharyngeal portion represent several maneuvers of the tongue in controlling exhaled air to form consonant sounds. A narrowly funneled stream of air made by the tongue striking and passing the teeth or alveolar ridge will produce a sound that is identified as a sibilant, or /s/. Adding phonation to this creates a voiced cognate, /z/. Elevating the posterior portion of the tongue to the soft palate and occluding the airway while exhaling causes a pause in air flow; when the tongue releases its contact with the velum, a /k/ or a voiced /g/ phone is produced. All of these, and most other consonants (except the nasals), require velopharyngeal closure. This affords oral air control without nasal air escape.

The anatomic structures in the mouth that act as *articulators* are discussed in Chapter 3. These are the upper and lower lips, the *oral vestibule* or sulcus between lips and teeth, and the bony *alveolar ridge.* The alveolar ridges are crescent-shaped bony structures that house teeth.

The teeth are also speech articulators. Biologically, they serve the purpose of mastication. The slicing incisor teeth, the tearing cuspids, the crushing bicuspids, and the pulverizing molars play their important roles in the mastication process.

Beyond the teeth, in the oral cavity proper, the walls are formed in part by the cheeks and the teeth. Within the cheeks are the two ducts providing some of the saliva to the mouth. Other sources of saliva are two glands beneath the tongue. The function of this fluid is to initiate the digestive process, to help dissolve food so that it can be tasted, to partly destroy bacteria in order to protect the oral mucosa, and to provide mucin to lubricate the bolus of food for swallowing.

The tongue itself is large enough to nearly fill the oral cavity. Its free anterior narrow portion, the apex or tip, is highly maneuverable in mastication and deglutition, as well as in speech articulation. On the under surface of the apex may be found a highly variable thin sheet of membrane, the *lingual frenulum* (frenum), at the midline from tongue to mouth floor.

Because all of his upper teeth were beyond the ability of a dentist to save by any means, Mr. Wong had them all extracted; he then moved through the several procedures for acquiring dentures. For Mr. Wong, as for all individuals, false teeth are a prosthesis requiring careful "custom fabrication" for the individual, his mouth, his sensitivities, his habits, and his preferences. After several visits, Mr. Wong's upper denture was delivered. It fit extremely well, and his new teeth were cosmetically ideal. However, he found a new problem: his speech. The /s/ and /z/ and /ʃ/ sounds were "slushy," he said, and made his speech difficult to understand; they attracted undue attention. A speech pathologist found that perhaps because he had lost some of the space for lingual touch, because the surface of the denture plate was extremely smooth and polished, and because saliva made that surface slippery, Mr. Wong had problems in lingual placement for articulation. The speech pathologist had small "bumps" placed on the denture and taught Mr. Wong about articulation, with encouraging results.

The tongue dorsum rests near the palate, which is the ceiling of the oral cavity. The palate also forms the floor of the nasal passages, so it is a *septum* (wall) between the two chambers. It is an arched ceiling, varying considerably from person to person in the degree and form of its arching. The bony ceiling of the oral cavity is continued backward by the *soft palate* or *velum.*

The soft palate slopes downward and backward, terminating in the vestigial *uvula,* a highly variable structure. The soft palate itself is largely musculature. The muscles contract to elevate and retract the velum in the important action of velopharyngeal closure during deglutition and speaking (Fig. 7.5). Recall that the term "velopharyngeal" refers to both soft palate and pharynx. To close off the nasopharynx (and nose) during swallowing and speech requires contraction of muscles of the velum and the pharynx together. Other muscles depress the soft palate to return the system to patency for nasal breathing.

The hypernasality in her voice bothered not only Melissa but her parents and her preschool teacher, among others. Nasal air escape also weakened the oral production of consonants. Melissa's speech was becoming quite difficult to understand and was distinctly "different." Evaluation by a physician and a speech pathologist failed to identify an anatomic problem, such as a cleft palate. The soft palate was quite active during speech. Close inspection of the pharyngeal walls, by visual as well as x-ray means, showed that the side walls of the pharynx were nearly completely immobile. No reason could be found for this, but the effect was clear: velopharyngeal closure during speech was very incompetent. A prosthodontist examined Melissa, agreed on the findings, and commenced building a prosthesis that would fit into Melissa's pharynx. It was immediately effective; the soft palate swung into a closure position against the prosthesis. Happily, over time, the prosthesis stimulated the sluggish pharyngeal muscles into action. It was possible later to remove the prosthesis; a plastic surgeon operated on Melissa to attach a pharyngeal flap across the pharynx, and her speech showed good potential without the prosthesis. Speech training then became quite effective in improving her oral communication.

Although of little importance to most speech and swallowing activities, the nasal passageways serve other important functions. Certainly, breathing is primary. Nasal breathing serves to warm, moisten, and filter incoming environmental air. The upper regions of the nasal passages also house sensory end organs for *olfaction,* the sense of smell.

AGING

As the individual reaches adulthood, structural changes lead to functional changes. The reverse is also true: not only does function follow structure, but structure follows function. In other words, use or disuse has an effect upon the form of the body.

Changes induced naturally, perhaps genetically, are called "aging processes." When they start varies considerably; perhaps genetic influences apply here. It has been said, facetiously, that one begins to age immediately after birth. Aging is simply the process of maturation, sometimes beyond the desirable levels. In fact, one demonstration of the aging process is found in the anatomy of the nervous system. This system commonly starts with perhaps more than 10 billion nerve cells. As we age, we lose on the average about 100 thousand such cells daily. Some persons lose more nerve cells more rapidly and earlier than others. The vocal tract is as susceptible to aging differences as are other body areas.

Although it may be difficult to separate "natural" aging changes from those that are encouraged by deleterious body-care habits, by injury, or by disease, some changes are termed "degenerative." These may be considered "natural" changes by some, but to the person who is undergoing such changes they may be viewed quite differently. Such changes include loss of teeth; changes in mucous membranes, muscle strength and responsiveness, and bone strength; difficulties with the joints such as in arthritis; and so on. To repeat, changes in the aging process are certainly natural processes, but may be undesirable to the individual in whom the changes are occurring.

Mr. Ashton has had increasingly difficult experiences in a number of areas because of his increasingly severe Parkinson's disease. This "shaking palsy" has affected much of his fine motor skills. His ability to write, his hobby of carving, even his handling of his knife and fork have all suffered as this central nervous system defect affects much of his everyday activities. This is very noticeable in his speech, even though his language skills remain fairly intact. The articulation is less precise, his voice shows a tremor and "flatness," and his vocal quality has lost its old ring. All of these decreased abilities leave Mr. Ashton feeling incapable, helpless, and at times even angry.

Summary of Anatophysiology and Development

The anatomic regions described above serve the important functions involved in mastication, deglutition, and respiration; they are also important in speech production. Persons may also be interested in facial appearance, which is affected by these structures. Such an interest commences in childhood and very probably continues throughout life. The development of these structures begins prenatally in the embryo, continuing through the fetal period to childhood and beyond. Some communication disorders stem from malformations occurring during the first months of gestation.

In this review of anatomy and physiology of the vocal tract and the development and maturation process, those structures, spaces, and functions involved in speech disorders have been deliberately highlighted. What areas of speech production are involved in such disorders?

REVIEW OF SPEECH PRODUCTION

Starting at the lowermost aspect of the vocal tract, we will first examine the phonatory system and the energy source for phonation, the air supply. Phonation is an aerodynamic, myoelastic phenomenon. The exhaled air from the lungs supplies the energy to vibrate the approximated vocal folds. The air flow and pressure vibrate the folds, but only when they are brought into juxtaposition will sound be produced. Depending upon the frequency (or pitch) the speaker desires, the folds are stretched or shortened, placed into tense or lax condition, thickened or thinned by muscular contractions.

The laryngeal tone is delivered into resonance chambers. The vestibule of the larynx, the laryngopharynx, the oropharynx, and the oral cavity are among those commonly used as resonance chambers. Resonance then takes place in adjustable anatomic chambers. They may be coupled, as in nasal sounds, so that the nasopharynx and nasal passages are added to the vocal resonance system. Some languages, such as French and Portuguese, have more nasalized sounds than does English. Though there might be general identity in the anatomy of the resonating chambers, they are used differently by different persons in different languages.

The maneuverability of the walls and the constricting mechanisms become extremely important to the nature of the acoustic product, the voice. The neural control to the muscles, the nature of the muscles themselves, the character of the surface membranes, the contour or shape of the walls of the various chambers, and the volumes of the cavities are among the elements that contribute to the resonance of the voice. It is these that one pays attention to when identifying a resonance disorder.

Still more is accomplished by the upper vocal tract. Articulation is an immediately observable event in speech. The articulators listed and described earlier are the structural elements that act to form the vowels and consonants of speech. Vowels are described as high and low, front and back, determined physiologically by the posture of the tongue in the resonating chamber: the mouth. Stops, fricatives, affricates, glides, and nasal consonants are used as acoustic descriptions of phonemes that are produced by the articulators. Phonation is also involved because so many speech-sounds are voiced.

The vocal tract is very forgiving. Many times persons have problems with the articulators that do not seriously affect the production of speech-sounds. A child who loses one or more teeth need not have an articulation disorder, although it is not unknown for this to happen. Instead, compensatory maneuvers utilize alternative articulatory activities to produce acceptable speech-sounds. But there are indeed several types of anatomic and physiologic differences that interfere with speech production. Keep in mind that some of the disorders create biologic dysfunction as well as speech problems. Some speech-language pathologists find themselves just as involved with resolving problems in these underlying biologic functions as they are in dealing with the communication disorders. What are some of the organic problems that one may find?

COMMON ANATOPHYSIOLOGIC DEFECTS ASSOCIATED WITH SPEECH DISORDERS

Speech pathologists have traditionally been serving individuals with *cleft palate* for many years. The anatomic defect that underlies the speech disorder occurs during embryonic development. The separate palatal shelves should have fused to wall off the nasal from the oral cavities. Some individuals have a cleft lip (on one or both sides of the upper lip) or varying degrees of clefts in the facial areas and even in the cranial region. Some of these defects stem from genetic anomalies. In other cases, the clefting condition may stem from biochemical or other influences upon the embryo. Failure of the tongue to lower from between the palatal shelves may prevent the palate from closing in some cases.

Whatever the cause, the infant may be born with the nasal passage coupled with the oral cavity through the unfused bony or soft palate. The cleft palate can cause a number of difficulties in the infant. First and most important, at this or any time, is the ability of the child to be nourished. Food entering the oral cavity can as freely pass into the nose as it can into the pharynx and thus the digestive tract. Getting the child to thrive is indeed a first priority.

Second, it is not entirely healthy for nasal and oral secretions to pass freely from one cavity to the other. Among the problems is the location of the auditory (Eustachian) tube leading to the middle ear. Also, displaced muscles may fail to ventilate and drain the ear as they should. Foreign materials (e.g., milk) could enter the tube to the ear.

Third, in the case of any accompanying cleft lip, the appearance of the youngster can be a problem. The facial appearance of a child with a cleft lip might adversely affect a relationship with other persons.

Lastly, a cleft palate can create abnormal speech patterns. If the cleft is left open, the child has a decreased ability to maintain air flow and pressure in the oral cavity, and there is no way of restricting resonance to that cavity. The result of these failures creates two possibilities. One is that the child is unable to articulate the pressure sounds of speech: the stops, affricates, and fricatives. The air needed by the oral structures to form these sounds has escaped into the nose and is lost for articulation. It can be lost completely causing articulatory omissions, or it can be weakened causing articulatory distortions (Fig. 7.6). The second possibility is that the resonated laryngeal tone is also unrestrained from entering the nasopharynx and the nasal passages. A nasal resonance is added to the vocal quality. This abnormal nasal resonance, or *hypernasality,* occurs in varying degrees from minimal to severe, from barely observable to making speech unintelligible.

These two characteristics of speech that can result from cleft palate may stem not only from frank cleft palate, but from other conditions as well. One is a close relative to the open cleft: an occult or hidden cleft palate. In this case, the palatal shelves again have failed to fuse, but the mucous membranes that line the oral cavity manage to bridge the gap. Apparently, and only apparently, the palate is intact. The effects can be as disordered as in a more common open cleft palate. The same evaluation and treatment procedures may be utilized for the one as for the other.

Robert developed hypernasality and nasal air emission at the age of about nine years. It came upon him after he had his tonsils and adenoids removed as a treatment for repeated sore throats and ear infections. However, the expected nasal quality that often

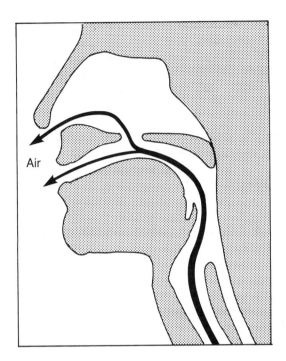

Figure 7.6.   Schematic of Cleft Palate Air Flow in Speech

occurs after adenoids are removed did not "go away" as usually happens. Not only did his voice have its unusual and undesirable nasal resonance but his speech was difficult to understand. Careful examination of the oral and pharyngeal anatomy did not show a cleft palate or any paralysis. Even more careful examination, however, showed a slight depression in the middle of the soft palate that was slightly bluish in color. There was also a *bifid* (split) uvula. These signs in the presence of the speech problems strongly suggested a submucous cleft palate, which is hidden or occult because the cleft itself is covered by mucous membrane. A plastic surgeon was called upon by the speech pathologist. Closure of the cleft, along with slight revision in the length of the soft palate, resulted in a much improved potential for good speech.

Another organic basis for hypernasality and/or nasal air emission is *paralysis or paresis of the velopharyngeal closure system*. This was noted in Chapter 5, and it is useful to repeat some aspects of the problem here. Neurogenic disorders may stem from degenerative pathologies of the nervous system, such as myasthenia gravis or amyotrophic lateral sclerosis, or they may be associated with the aging process. A neurogenic disorder may originate from a brain injury that disables the central brain regions or the peripheral nerves serving the velopharyngeal closure system. Such a disorder can result from physical trauma, a penetrating wound, or an extensive

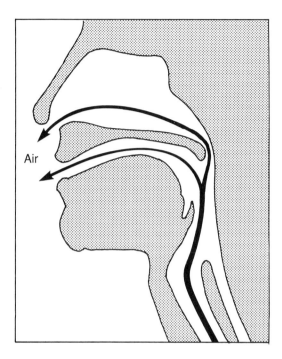

Figure 7.7. Schematic of Paralyzed Palate Air Flow in Speech

surgical procedure (such as removal of a cancerous growth from the pharyngeal region). Alternatively, a cerebral vascular accident (stroke) or other brain abnormality may initiate the disorder (Fig. 7.7).

The speech disorder is characterized by *nasal air escape* and resulting consonant weakness or omission. Hypernasality is present. These point to velopharyngeal closure problems of some type. A close examination of this system by a speech-language pathologist may well disclose the anatomic basis and lead to appropriate management. Such management may lie in the province of a specialist in another field: surgery or dentistry, for example.

Speech disorders may be associated with other structural defects of the oral cavity. A common one not usually attended by the speech pathology profession is that stemming from *the edentulous state.* When for some reason a person loses teeth, especially the upper teeth, speech problems may result. In most cases, the person compensates for the loss, and whatever speech differences arise may be minimal. Yet, significant and important speech problems do develop in some cases.

The specialist associated with dentures, as well as other prosthetic appliances for defects of the oral cavity, is the *prosthodontist.* General dentists who have studied and practiced in this area also occasionally make prostheses. Dentures, colloquially called false teeth, are carefully designed for the patient's own oral cavity. Dentures consist of teeth that are artificially embedded in a plastic resin or acrylic material. Upper dentures also have a plate that covers at least the bony palate. With the help of adhesives, such dentures adhere fairly well to the palate throughout the day. In contrast, however, dentures for the lower arch adhere less well because they cannot cover the same surface area (the intervening tongue prevents this). Fortunately, lower denture problems are not often associated with speech problems. In either case, upper or lower, dentures may be better fitted with implanted pins to which the prosthesis is attached. Articulation problems may occur, especially with upper dentures. "Whistling" /s/, "slushy" articulation, "muffled" speech—all sometimes describe the speech of persons having difficulties with these dentures. Speech pathologists often have assistive remedies, or at least ameliorating approaches, for many of these problems.

A few defects occurring in the tongue may relate to speech disorders. *Paralysis of the tongue muscles, tongue-tie,* and *surgical excision* of parts of the tongue may be the most commonly encountered.

Paralysis of the tongue may be on one side or both (unilateral or bilateral), depending upon the place of damage to the nervous system. Either would have its consequences in the tongue's ability to form the constrictions necessary for consonant production and to make delicate maneuvers in creating a vowel-resonating space. At times, the speech-language pathologist might be able to stimulate increased lingual function, develop compensatory articulatory maneuvers, or work with the prosthodontist in creating a prosthesis to assist in both speaking and eating. A surgical specialist may sometimes be consulted to make structural changes that might improve tongue behaviors. There is no universally accepted approach because so very many different kinds and degrees of tongue paralyses exist.

A tongue-tie, as discussed in Chapter 3, occurs when the lingual frenum limits the mobility of the tongue apex. As one might expect, there are differing degrees of severity of tongue-tie. It is not a common defect. When the tongue apex is prevented from elevating in speech production (as in /s/, /l/, /t/, and other apical sounds) one might expect distortions to occur. Exercises are not usually given in such cases. Sometimes pharmaceuticals are injected into the region to soften and loosen the tissues. In other cases, a plastic surgeon might make a zig-zag cut into the frenum, freeing it and inhibiting regrowth (regrowth occasionally occurs when the frenum is simply clipped). Once the tongue apex is freed, speech-language pathologists often give the child minimal exercises in elevation and speech production, depending upon the nature of the associated speech disorder.

Some persons, usually adults, are found to have *abnormal growths* in or around the tongue region. The growths may be *benign* or *malignant.* The first term suggests that they do not spread elsewhere in the body, even though as growths they can present important problems to the patient. Malignant growths are a more extensive type of problem, one that can spread beyond its origin; it is more frequently identified as cancer. In either case, it might be the judgment of a medical practitioner and the patient to surgically remove the growth. Surgical removal of some part of the tongue is a *glossectomy.* Surgery extent varies, from a small portion, leaving little residual defect in structure or function, to a larger, e.g., a hemiglossectomy, involving a major part of the tongue. In some cases, the majority of the tongue may be removed (a *total glossectomy*), leaving the patient with considerable difficulties in chewing, swallowing, and speech. Reconstructive surgeries and lingual prostheses may be considered, along with the assistance of a speech-language pathologist.

A behavior that may be related to disordered speech is *tongue-thrust.* This term refers to a forward positioning of the tongue. Some deny that this is a speech-related disorder because the basic clinical research is sparse and sometimes equivocal.[1] This claim is countered by other professionals who base their opinions on clinical experience and believe that tongue-thrust is an important biologic dysfunction that can be remediated by appropriate techniques. Many speech-language pathologists associate some articulation disorders with this behavior and manage or remediate accordingly. Another group of professionals—dentists, usually orthodontists—regard tongue-thrust as important to teeth; they may refer their patients to speech-language pathologists for clinical management. Others employ special devices in the mouth with the intention of forcing the tongue into other than tongue-thrust behaviors. What is this behavior that is called tongue-thrusting and why is it considered a problem?

The forward posturing of the tongue can be quite variable. It can be forward during any of three activities: in the resting position, during swallowing activities, and in speech behaviors. The tongue apex can be observed against the anterior teeth or even protruding between the upper and lower teeth. It is also claimed that it may be placed against or through the teeth at the sides of the mouth. The speech results commonly are sibilant distortions, a form of protrusional lisp, among other effects.

> Molly was 17 when her dentist referred her to an orthodontist because her teeth were in malocclusion, an overbite and open bite. Besides that, Molly had had speech therapy for several years, primarily for sibilant distortion that "would not go away." The orthodontist examined her and among other things found that Molly had a strong anterior tongue-thrust, which was considered an underlying factor behind the dental malocclusion. The orthodontist referred her to a speech pathologist whose examination confirmed the opinion of the dentist, and speech training began. First, it approached the tongue placement in all behaviors. Then as Molly improved, emphasis was placed upon the speech difference. With decrease in the tongue-thrusting behavior in all activities and improvement in sibilant production, the orthodontist felt free to commence orthodontic treatment while the speech pathologist recalled Molly at about quarterly periods for evaluation and reinforcement of the improved speech she had gained.

Few speech problems are associated with the lips. Examples include disorders with a neuromotor etiology and cleft lip resulting from embryonic development failure. Occasionally a person may develop *facial paralysis,* usually unilaterally.

(1989) *ASHA* Vol. 31, Nov. 92 94. This report of a special ad-hoc committee concluded that therapy for tongue-thrusting and associated problems is appropriate and within the purview of speech-language pathology as long as pathologists are appropriately prepared and that research in these areas should continue.

Difficulty in closing the mouth firmly on one side may occur; this will be more evident because of uncontrollable drooling. Lip closure in some consonant sound productions could be affected. Sometimes such paralyses are transitory and the patient recovers full function with time. Otherwise, help from physicians and surgeons must be sought. Speech-language pathologists attempt to control saliva, train for muscle compensation, and work to remove any associated speech problems.

In the case of the child born with a *cleft lip*, unilateral or bilateral, complete or incomplete, a great variety of possible conditions and effects may take place. As the child develops, speech may have a few distortions, although in the case of a cleft lip alone (not associated with cleft palate or other problems) there are rarely major speech disorders. Because of two other problems, feeding and cosmesis, plastic surgery is often done within the first few weeks. When a cleft lip is associated with other defects such as cleft palate, then the lip surgery is but the first of a number of other procedures performed in the early years of life.

Problems stemming from the effects of cancer were mentioned previously. Glossectomy and laryngectomy are procedures performed to save the patient's life, but leave a speech problem to be resolved. Cancer also can be found elsewhere in the vocal tract. Lip and cheek cancers appear occasionally, especially in certain tobacco users. Cancer of the bones in the oral cavity region can develop. The palate and the pharynx may be invaded by the cells of the disease. And, of course, the larynx may be the site of life-threatening cancer growth; surgical laryngectomy is first a life-saving procedure. A patient with cancer, wherever it might be focused, is seriously threatened. Much research is in progress not only to find the various causes of the disease, but to discover more and better ways to remediate its effects.

Patients with cancer history are treated by a variety of means. Pharmaceutical agents of several types, depending upon the kind and location of the cancerous growth, are one approach. Such chemotherapy takes several forms and has several results. Another approach utilizes radiation therapy, either by radium or by special x-ray application. Again, the success rate depends heavily upon the type of cancer and its location in the body. Other approaches include surgical excision of the growth and associated anatomic tissues.

Removal by surgery of parts of the maxilla bone, the mandible bone, the soft palate, the hard palate, the epiglottis, and the larynx may be performed. As a result, chewing, swallowing, and speech problems (among others) may occur. Speech pathologists are among the helping professionals who might be involved in the return of the patient to better functioning. Improved articulation, resonance, and compensatory phonatory approaches fall under the aegis of these specialists.

Lastly, some of the *degenerative neurologic disorders* may leave the patient with a variety of important problems, among which may be a speech disorder. Language, too, is often a concern, especially in some of the problems accompanying senility, such as Alzheimer's disease. Not only do speech-language pathologists concern themselves with the speech and language difficulties of such patients, but often they assess and treat some of the more basic biologic disorders stemming from the same degenerative or other condition.

Speech-language pathologists may be called upon to assist patients with prob-lems of mastication as well as *deglutition* (swallowing). The latter disorders are termed *dysphagia.* Because of their knowledge of oral anatomy and physiology, speech-language pathologists might well be the best qualified at the scene to care for such patients. Using bedside assessment techniques and highly sophisticated radio-graphic approaches, such specialists can both identify such problems and direct therapeutic approaches designed to ameliorate them.

In other neurogenic speech disorders, as noted in Chapter 5, a patient may present with not only a speech disorder but a respiratory one. A patient who has a disease such as bulbar poliomyelitis, in which there is respiratory paralysis, must be placed on assistive breathing instruments (iron lungs, rocking beds, chest respira-tors). At times, a speech pathologists may be able to teach a rudimentary breathing technique known as glossopharyngeal or "frog" breathing. The patient learns to pump small bubbles of air into the airway in a sort of gulping fashion. This air can be maneuvered into the lungs. It is a backup or safeguard system for some patients and cannot always be used for everyday breathing. Respiratory therapists, of course, also teach glossopharyngeal breathing.

EVALUATION

Persons with speech-language disorders associated with anatomic and/or physi-ologic defects are often evaluated by a multidisciplinary group of specialists, including the speech-language pathologist. The nature of the specialties involved is dictated by the general nature of the defect. For example, in the case a child with a cleft palate, the pediatrician might be the primary caregiver, and consulting in evaluation and planning will be the plastic surgeon, a dental specialist, an ear-nose-throat physician, an audiolo-gist, a geneticist, and of course the speech-language pathologist.

Similar special "teams" are formed for other anatomic and physiologic disorders, a part of which might be oral communication disorders. A cancer (or oncology) team, a special neurologic disorders team, and so on, may be formed. These are discussed in greater detail in Chapter 10, which presents information about the nature of multi-disciplinary evaluation and treatment groups.

As discussed below, speech-language pathologists are increasingly found in medical centers of various types, serving with medical and dental specialists in their concern for the patients with anatomic speech disorders. Many larger hospitals and clinics provide the services of a communication specialist in evaluation procedures as well as in remediation approaches.

GENERAL MANAGEMENT APPROACHES: THE SPEECH-LANGUAGE PATHOLOGIST

It is beyond the scope of this chapter to present the techniques used in either evaluation or management for the multitude of differing anatomicophysiologic disor-ders of speech, the range of which should be clear from the wide gamut of differing problems discussed above. To use one illustration, the treatment for swallowing disorders requires very different approaches from those used for speech problems stemming from cleft palate. There may well be overlapping or perhaps similar aspects in other disorders. For example, swallowing disorders may occur in both neurogenic and cancer surgery patients, with their widely differing etiologies.

Management consists of specialized approaches to a particular patient with a particular problem. The speech-language pathologist determines the nature of the speech disorder, identifies etiologic conditions, examines possible avenues to follow in remediation, calls in associated specialists to assist in offering therapeutic approaches, and monitors changes in the patient as the work progresses. It is a dramatic, important, still-developing practice arena for the professional in speech-language pathology.

Clearly, speech-language pathologists may find themselves in a fair number of situations involving patients with anatomic and physiologic disorders. The necessary specialists are called upon to evaluate, offer planning, and perform procedures that will help the patient through and past his/her problems to the highest levels of function possible. As noted above, the majority of such patients with extensive disorders in several physiologic realms are cared for by teams of specialists, including speech-language pathologists. At times, such teams are formed for a particular patient. At other times, as is often found in the field of cleft palate, teams that have been functioning together for some time serve a number of patients.

Some speech-language pathologists may be more experienced in working with patients having anatomically based speech disorders. Most of these professionals will be serving in medically oriented situations such as hospitals and rehabilitation centers. Although the basic or general educational preparation for these highly specialized speech-language pathologists differs little from that for speech-language pathologists serving children in school settings, the postgraduate and continuing education work of the more specialized professional will focus upon the anatomy-based disorders. In Chapter 10 we will describe the education and the accreditation of speech-language pathologists and audiologists.

SUMMARY

We have listed and described a number of defects and diseases that involve anatomic and physiologic systems and may concurrently lessen speech skills. There has been no attempt to be exhaustive in such coverage; for example, we have not directly discussed the infinitely variable defects that might arise from automobile accidents, war wounds, and injuries sustained anywhere in everyday life. Genetic influences create a large number of what are known as craniofacial deformities for which heroic surgeries and highly individual remediation approaches must be devised. Defects originating in embryonic formation differences and degenerative neurologic conditions often underlie the oral communication disorder with which the speech-language pathologist may have to deal.

SUGGESTED READINGS

This chapter is unusual in that its subject matter involves medical, dental, anatomic, and other special fields. Further reading material may be found in a medical school library or in your own physician's or dentist's library. There are some general references that will allow you to acquire a more thorough and perhaps more clear idea of the matters discussed. First, some gross anatomy texts. The latest editions are given here, but any earlier edition will suffice.

Anson, B. J. (Ed.) (1966). *Human Anatomy: A Complete Systematic Treatise,* 12th ed. New York: McGraw-Hill. (Also known as *Morris' Human Anatomy.*)

Clemente, C. D. (Ed.) (1985). *Anatomy of the Human Body by Henry Gray,* 30th ed. Philadelphia: Lea & Febiger. *Over a thousand pages of detailed text with a large number of illustrations presenting the anatomy of the entire body. It is the most commonly known anatomy text to the general public.*

Romanes, G. J. (Ed.) (1981). *Cunningham's Textbook of Anatomy,* 12th ed. Oxford/New York: Oxford University Press.

Anatomic atlases are excellent picture books, with minimal text or descriptive information. The following is an old favorite, but there are several others you may find useful.

Anderson, J. E. (Ed.) (1983). *Grant's Atlas of Anatomy,* 8th ed. Baltimore: Williams & Wilkins.

The gross anatomy texts provide details of human development. Physiology texts will also describe this important period in the development of the human body. We recommend in particular:

Tortora, G. J., and N. K. Anagnostakos (1990). *Principles of Anatomy and Physiology,* 6th ed. New York: Harper & Row. *Embryology is presented in Chapter 25 with very helpful highlighting of interesting and important areas.*

In the field of communication disorders, several speech scientists have prepared anatomic and physiologic texts of considerable value:

Kahane, J. C., and J. F. Folkins (1984). *Atlas of Speech and Hearing Anatomy.* Columbus, OH: Charles E. Merrill. *A photographic atlas, in the main, with little descriptive materials. The photographs are exceptionally clear, however.*

Kaplan, H. (1971). *Anatomy and Physiology of Speech,* 2nd ed. New York: McGraw-Hill. *Another carefully crafted and detailed anatomy and physiology text.*

Palmer, J. (1984). *Anatomy for Speech and Hearing,* 3rd ed. New York Harper & Row. *A narrowly focused anatomy text with deemphasis of physiology and speech production.*

Perkins, W., and R. Kent (1986). *Functional Anatomy of Speech, Language, and Hearing: A Primer.* San Diego: College Hill Press. *A useful primer of anatomy having a combination of simplified descriptive matter, line drawings of narrowly focused areas, self-study devices, and emphasis upon the functional.*

Zemlin, W. (1981). *Speech and Hearing Sciences,* 2nd ed. Englewood Cliffs, NJ: Prentice-Hall. *Probably the best-known text in its field. It has ample discussion of physiology and anatomy; acoustics and aerodynamics as well as speech production are well described.*

Texts on speech disorders emphasizing problems with anatophysiologic bases are not common, but a few are important:

Bzoch, K. (1979). *Communicative Disorders Related to Cleft Palate,* 2nd ed. Boston: Little, Brown & Co. *A selection of focused chapters from a larger text that includes much of interest to surgeons, dentists, geneticists, and the like. Both books provide much information helpful to the student of speech pathology.*

Groher, M. (Ed.) (1984). *Dysphagia: Diagnosis and Management.* Stoneham, MA: Butterworth. *A highly specialized text concerned with swallowing problems, edited by a speech pathologist and directed toward such professionals.*

Logemann, J. A. (1983). *Swallowing Disorders*. San Diego: College Hill Press. *Detailed information concerning the various aspects of swallowing problems, and detailed descriptions of performing and using radiographic studies.*

McWilliams, B. J., H. Morris, and R. Shelton (1984). *Cleft Palate Speech*. St. Louis: C. V. Mosby. *A thorough compendium of the embryology, anatomy, physiology, speech, and assessment, and therapy of the patient with cleft lip and cleft palate.*

Wells, C. (1971). *Cleft Palate and Its Associated Speech Disorders*. New York: McGraw-Hill. *A somewhat older text, but with some thorough discussions of etiologies and therapies as well as other aspects of cleft palate.*

Other areas for which texts of a specialized nature are available include the cerebral palsies, aphasia, dysarthria, and tongue-thrust. Students are encouraged to seek out as many specialized texts as their interests dictate.

Study Questions

1. Describe at least two different anatomic or physiologic problems underlying hypernasality and distorted (weakened) consonant sound productions.

2. How would you associate degree of injury to (or loss of) the tongue with degree of speech impairment?

3. How do you think it might be possible to damage the nerves leading to the muscles of phonation, resonance, and articulation?

4. Swallowing problems may be associated with several different anatomic defects; can you identify three?

5. A speech-language pathologist, when seeing a patient with an anatomic problem, is often forced to refer to other specialists. Identify three such non-speech specialists and the anatomic problems with which they deal that would also involve a speech pathologist.

6. Look up in a medical textbook, or ask your instructor or your physician, what effects on speech might result from enlarged adenoids.

7. In your own experience, what speech problems develop when a child (aged five to eight years) loses some of his/her teeth?

8. Speech and language disorders often stem from brain injury. List several other life problems suffered by a person with a brain injury. Can you list some sort of priority for caring for these problems? What bases do you use for such a ranking?

9. Do you think it would be difficult to differentiate between a person who does not understand spoken language because of brain injury and a person who has an important hearing impairment? Without looking up standardized tests and procedures, how could you make a first guess?

10. What is the relevence of muscle training to speech therapy? What kinds of disorders might be treated using this as one of the approaches?

8

The Normal and the Impaired Ear

The sea of sound in which we live offers innumerable opportunities for contact with the surrounding world. Our visual impressions are constantly enhanced by associated auditory stimulation. Even without sight, sound still provides a wealth of information about the environment: door chimes or a telephone bell two rooms away; a hungry baby in a crib upstairs; the emergent message of an approaching siren—all are examples of important signals in our lives that would be unknown to us without hearing.

From time to time we may prefer silence over the invasive nature of some sounds, whether barely audible (a dripping faucet on a sleepless night) or extremely loud (industrial noise so loud even our shouts cannot be understood). For the hearing, choices can be made. Earplugs can be worn to cope with unwanted sound, and speech comprehension can still be preserved. But for the hearing impaired, simply making sound louder rarely leads to the rich auditory experiences enjoyed by the normally hearing.

The causes and human consequences of hearing impairment will be discussed in this and the following chapter. We will explore ways in which hearing loss is managed by the physician, the audiologist, the hearing aid specialist, the teacher of the hearing impaired, and others. But before we can adequately address these topics, a fundamental understanding of the normal ear and how it functions is essential. We must know how sound is typically processed before we can fully grasp the implications of disordered hearing.

PROCESSING AUDITORY SIGNALS

The sounds we hear are composed of rapidly changing physical events occurring every fraction of a second. Although they often arise within our immediate environment, some sounds originating from considerable distances can still be perceived. The sound source must be something capable of vibrating, such as the diaphragm of a loudspeaker or a person's vocal folds. These vibrations reach our ears as the energy at the source is carried outward from molecule to molecule within the surrounding air. As detailed in Chapter 4, we characterize these events in terms of the number of times they occur each second (the *frequency* of the sound, measured in *Hertz*) and their relative energy at any point in time (the *intensity*, in *decibels*). Remember the abbreviations for these two terms: Hz and dB.

It is the function of the ear to convert these acoustic signals into a stimulus that is recognized by the listener as sound. This is not a simple task. The frequencies and intensities of sound are extremely variable over time and highly complex in their spectral characteristics. Correct judgments depend on extremely high fidelity within the listening apparatus. The normally operating auditory system is exquisite in its function, responding instantaneously to intricate signal variations that often change each millisecond, transforming an acoustic incident into a mechanical event, and finally into actions within the nervous system. This activity, often referred to as *auditory processing*, results in a psychologic impression that the listener characterizes as "pitch," "loudness," "noise," "speech," "music," etc.

THE AUDITORY MECHANISM

The recognition of sound as a stimulus worthy of our attention cannot begin until the auditory area of the brain perceives a signal from one or both ears. Three major processes must occur:

1. Airborne sound pressures entering the ear canal must be transformed into mechanical vibrations of tiny bones and membranes in the middle and inner ears.
2. This energy must then be converted into activity within the central nervous system and reach the auditory area of the brain.
3. The stimulus must be processed so that it is recognized by the listener as auditory information.

These three stages occur in the above sequence and with incredible speed. They operate constantly throughout our lives. If the energy of sound that surrounds us is sufficient, this complex mechanical and electrochemical transmission process occurs whether we are asleep or awake, 24 hours a day. The third stage, auditory perception, depends on our state of attentiveness. Although the chances of hearing during a deep sleep are obviously remote, we can be equally unaware of the auditory stimulus when awake if our attention is focused elsewhere.

The steps described are closely related to specific structures within the auditory system. Figures 8.1 and 8.2 are cross-sections of the right ear, drawn as if the skull were parted at a line between the right and left ear and the front half were removed to reveal the ear's interior. Note that the acoustic stimulus from surrounding air must travel through four structural parts: the outer, the middle, and the inner ears, and the auditory nervous system. As it traverses this pathway, the physical signal is transformed into mechanical vibrations and, in turn, into nerve energy that eventually

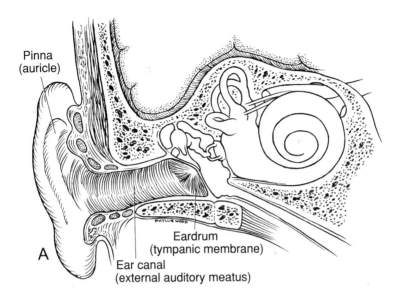

A

Pinna
(auricle)

Eardrum
(tympanic membrane)

Ear canal
(external auditory meatus)

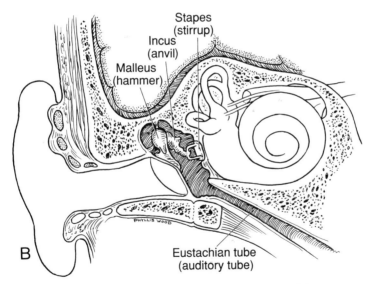

B

Stapes
(stirrup)

Incus
(anvil)

Malleus
(hammer)

Eustachian tube
(auditory tube)

Figure 8.1. Views of the Outer Ear (A) and the Middle Ear (B)
Cross-section of the right temporal bone, showing the major components of the conductive system.

stimulates the brain. Let us examine these intricate processes as they occur within the auditory system.

The Outer Ear

The primary function of the outermost portion of the ear is to provide an initial pathway for transmission of the airborne acoustic signal into the head. The visible appendage located immediately behind the canal opening (Fig. 8.1A) is well known to us. The *pinna*, or *auricle*, is of considerable importance to the hearing of certain animal species that have exceptional muscular control of the structure. By moving each pinna independently, these animals can more efficiently direct into the canal opening high-frequency sounds that are inaudible to the human ear. These species (such as bats, horses, cats, and certain dogs) generally have far better sensitivity for such sounds than do humans.

The *ear canal* (external auditory meatus) is the primary conduit for airborne sound to reach the *eardrum* (tympanic membrane). This is a tough, multilayered structure situated at the end of the canal. It forms the boundary between the outer and middle ears. Functionally, however, it is a part of the middle ear. The membrane is normally so thin that structures in the middle-ear cavity can often be observed by looking into the ear canal with a strong light.

The Middle Ear

This portion of the ear is a small, air-filled cavity situated internal to the tympanic membrane (Fig. 8.1B). Normally, the air pressure inside the middle ear is the same as that which surrounds us. This condition is maintained by periodic openings of the *Eustachian* (auditory) *tube*, which in adults extends downward from the middle ear to the back of the nasopharynx. Although the tube is normally closed, muscular movements during swallowing and yawning may open it momentarily. In this way, the air pressure on both sides of the membrane is instantly equalized. This allows the membrane to be maximally compliant when sound waves passing along the ear canal finally make contact, since it is in its natural position.

What if the middle-ear pressure is significantly different from that in the ear canal and the surrounding environment? If it is less, the eardrum will be pushed in by the higher pressure in the canal. If the pressure is higher in the middle ear, the membrane will be displaced outward. In either case, the eardrum will be abnormally stretched and stiffened, making it less responsive to weak acoustic pressure changes. The normal function of the auditory tube, therefore, is vital in maintaining the natural status of the tympanic membrane.

The sound energy moving the tympanic membrane must be conveyed quickly and efficiently into the sensory mechanism of the ear. This is accomplished by setting into vibration a chain of three tiny bones, called the *ossicles*. These bones form a bridge across the middle-ear space, directly connecting the tympanic membrane with an opening into the inner ear (the *oval window*, Fig. 8.2). Sometimes referred to as the hammer, anvil, and stirrup, the ossicles are known anatomically as the *malleus, incus,* and *stapes* (Fig. 8.1*B*). The handle of the malleus is embedded securely within the fibrous layer of the tympanic membrane so that this bone, as well as the two to which it is attached, will move in response to the membrane's vibrations. The ossicles are delicately balanced in the middle-ear space by an intricate system of ligaments and two tiny muscles. Consequently, the entire mechanism is normally responsive to minute vibrations of the membrane. For what purpose is this transmission process built into our ears? Why does sound not simply travel directly from the tympanic membrane into the inner ear without having to pass through this complicated mechanical system?

There are several reasons. The most important, by far, is the need to transfer sound energy from the gaseous medium of environmental air into the much denser fluid filling the inner ear, where the auditory nerve is stimulated. The high opposition, or *impedance,* to particle movement found in this liquid medium must somehow be matched efficiently with the relatively unimpeded transmission of sound energy occurring in air. If not, most of the energy entering the ear would be reflected back from the openings into the inner ear. The ossicular system provides the answer. It operates as a high-fidelity "transformer." This important mechanical function is accomplished by essentially "focusing" the energy vibrating the tympanic membrane into the smaller area of the oval window at the base of the stapes. In addition, the ossicles operate as a mechanical lever, adding more efficiency to the transformer function. These actions result in creating a force per unit area at the stapes footplate that is about 22 times greater than at the tympanic membrane. This extra force compensates for the higher resistance to the flow of energy in the cochlea.

As the footplate of the stapes rocks in and out of the oval window, the air-to-liquid transfer of sound energy finally occurs. The high impedance of the fluids compared with that of air is essentially compensated for by the efficient operation of the middle-ear transformer. Vibratory energy now enters the third part of the ear.

The Inner Ear

Like the middle ear and its contents, the inner ear occupies space created in the hardest bone of the body, the *temporal bone.* The walls of this structure, called the *cochlea,* are shaped something like a snail shell with about 2¹/₂ spirals (Fig. 8.2). The cochlea is divided into three compartments (scalae). As noted above, each of these spaces is fluid-filled. The upper and lower portions are continuous at the top, or apex, so they contain the same fluid (*perilymph*). Each of these chambers is terminated with a membranous "window" separating the cochlea from the middle ear. One is the oval window, discussed above. The other opening, located just below the oval window, is called the *round window.* Movements of the round window occur in response to stapedial vibrations at the oval window, thereby allowing sound energy to be exchanged within the fluid-filled spaces of the cochlea. Without the round window, energy entering the oval window would go nowhere since fluids in a closed space are relatively incompressible. This second window membrane provides the reciprocal "release valve" that is necessary for energy transfer within the cochlea. As the stapes

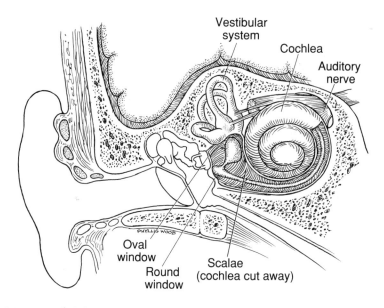

Figure 8.2.   View of the Inner Ear
Cross-section of the right ear, emphasizing the structure of the auditory and vestibular sensorineural systems.

moves in and out, energy is instantaneously transferred to the cochlear fluids and membranes. Since fluids cannot be compressed easily, this energy exchange could not occur without some outlet in the system releasing fluid pressure waves. This is provided by the round window.

And what of the middle portion of the cochlea's three-compartment system, which is also filled with fluid (*endolymph*)? This chamber contains the specialized receptor organ designed to activate the auditory nerve and send the stimulus to the brain. Arrayed from the base to the apex of the cochlea, this structure is named after the Italian count who was one of the first to describe its intricate anatomy (Alphonse de Corti). The *organ of Corti* contains about 23,000 microscopic sensory *hair cells* overlayed with a thin, gelatinous membrane. These cells are capable of direct contact with the membrane through delicate groups of hairs, or *cilia*, extending from their top surfaces. Some individual cells have up to 150 of these cilia.

The process by which certain of these sensory hair cells are stimulated by sound is really a continuation of the mechanical events reviewed thus far. As the stapes rocks back and forth in the oval window, corresponding waves of energy flow through the fluid just behind the oval window. This energy passes swiftly through the cochlea in specific patterns, depending primarily on the frequency and intensity of the sound, and therefore of stapes movement. Variations in stiffness and mass along the cochlea distribute the ease of membrane movement relative to the driving frequency. The membrane on which the organ of Corti sits is narrower and stiffer at the base, for example, becoming increasingly wider and more elastic as it gets closer to the apex. Consequently, this membrane and its associated end organ respond to tones of higher frequencies at the base and lower frequencies closer to the apex. The areas of maximum stimulation for intermediate frequencies are filtered and distributed in an orderly fashion between base and apex. This stimulation pattern, linking sound frequency with locus of activity in the auditory system, is critical to the brain's final determination of sound pitch.

As the cilia on the hair-cell surface are physically displaced, a complicated electrochemical process is initiated that stimulates the nerve ending at the base of the cell. It is at this point that the mechanical and vibratory activity ends. The stimulus now travels along the auditory nerve for transmission to the brain.

The Auditory Nervous System

The individual neurons and cell bodies associated with audition are organized into an intricate system extending from the cochlear hair cells to the auditory areas of the brain. The nerve fibers emerging from the cochlea join with those from the balance mechanism, the vestibular system. Although the organs associated with hearing and balance are closely approximated in the temporal bone, and even share the same fluid system, their function and neural connections remain quite independent.

The *vestibular system* keeps the brain informed of head position by the movement of fluid within three semicircular canals embedded in each of the two temporal bones (Fig. 8.2). These canals occur in three positional planes relative to the upright head: vertical, horizontal, and one that is somewhat oblique. Sensory cells are embedded at the base of each canal. As the head moves in a specific direction, the vestibular nerve is stimulated by physical movement patterns of specific cells in each of the two vestibular systems. These signals are combined in the central nervous system and are interpreted as a positional change according to learned response patterns.

The bundle of fibers emerging from each cochlea and vestibular system forms into cranial nerve VIII. The nerve passes through a tiny hole in the temporal bone and enters the skull cavity, where it connects with other neurons low in the brainstem. The number of neurons begins to increase as further interconnections occur in nuclei situated at higher levels. In this manner, the 25,000 fibers within the *auditory* portion of nerve VIII from each ear multiply to over a million neurons by the time the auditory cortex of the brain is reached.

Nerve activity from each ear combines in the brainstem to initiate binaural stimulation at the auditory cortex. Slight differences in the arrival times and intensities of signals reaching each ear independently are instantly compared and relayed to higher centers for analysis. These binaural cues are of great importance in localizing the source of a sound in our environment. At a very early stage we learn the position of interesting sounds in our surroundings by this instantaneous analysis of subtle variations in the acoustic signals arriving at our two ears.

Some neurons from each cochlea pass up the brainstem to the cortex on the same (ipsilateral) side. Most, however, cross over to the opposite (contralateral) side and enter the hemisphere on that side. Connections occur between both ascending tracks in the brainstem and even between the two hemispheres. Certain areas of the temporal cortex on each side of the brain are involved in audition, but the auditory cortex on only one side, usually the left, is predominantly responsible for the processing of speech. It is at the cortical level that the sensations within the nervous system are finally combined with impressions stored in memory, and auditory recognition can occur. The stimulus is heard at last!

The Air and Bone Pathways

Sound energy can reach the cochlear end organ through two major pathways. The first, *air conduction,* is the route normally used by airborne sound. Environmental stimuli are perceived through the pathway offering least resistance to its passage— the one providing the most efficient means by which energy can be transferred from gaseous to liquid media. The air-conduction route to the cochlea comprises the functional components of the outer and middle ears considered above. Since these two parts of the ear are involved in "conducting" airborne sound into the inner ear, they are often referred to as the *conductive* system. The remaining elements of the ear, composed of the sensory mechanism in the cochlea and the neural connections to the brain, are combined together into the *sensorineural* system. The air-conduction route encompasses both systems since it involves the outer, middle, and inner ears and the auditory nervous system.

There is another way for sound to enter the cochlea as well. This approach bypasses the outer and middle ears. Sound can be transmitted through the skull, using a pathway called *bone conduction.* Obviously such a route is highly inefficient compared with air conduction. The mass and stiffness of the skull bones require that the sound stimulus must be of a reasonably high intensity, or closely coupled to the head. Most surrounding airborne sound cannot meet this requirement.

> The viability of the bone-conduction pathway is best illustrated when we insert earplugs into one or both ears and note how our own vocalizations seem to be so much louder than before. Since the air-conduction pathway is now compromised by the plugs, we no longer hear the environmental noises around us. In a way, the cochlea is now in a quieter setting. The low-frequency vibrations from the larynx seem louder as we talk. We might also hear heart beats and digestive noises that we normally do not detect. Such sounds, rightfully so, are not a part of our typical sensation since the common environmental noises surrounding us are usually of sufficient intensity to "mask" them out of our perception.

AUDITORY PERCEPTION

Any explanation for how we hear must provide answers to many questions. Perhaps the most significant of these pertains to the perception of auditory pitch and loudness. How does this complex sensory system allow us to differentiate these familiar auditory impressions?

Pitch

As pointed out in the previous discussion of the mechanical action within the cochlea, certain areas of the cochlea are stimulated when specific acoustic frequencies enter the ear. A tone of a high frequency, say 4,000 Hertz (Hz), causes the tympanic membrane, ossicles, and oval window to move with the same number of vibratory movements each second. These movements, in turn, evoke membrane and fluid displacement in the cochlea that is concentrated primarily toward the base because of the sound's high frequency. Major activity at this position is governed primarily by membrane stiffness and mass and by the physical space occupied by the cochlear compartments. Both of these dimensions vary from base to apex.

Once the hair cells are stimulated in a specific area, impulses created in associated neurons convey a "message" to the brain that a sound of a high frequency has entered the ear. This occurs because of the sensitivity of individual nerve fibers as well as the interconnections between the cochlea and the auditory area of the brain.

Careful research on the neuroanatomy and physiology of the auditory system has revealed many interesting facts. Two are particularly relevant to this discussion. First, not all neurons respond equally to all sound frequencies. Certain neurons seem to be "tuned," responding to certain discrete frequencies and not to others. Some are activated more easily when stimulated a small number of times each second. Others will function only for signals of a higher frequency. But none of them can fire independently more than 2,000 times each second. How, then, can we hear sounds having frequencies much higher than this? A possible explanation is that individual neurons from a specific part of the basilar membrane may initiate their firing patterns at different times. The resulting "volleys" of a neuron group, when combined, appear to represent a higher frequency of stimulation by the time they reach the brain than would be the case for any individual neuron.

A second fact learned from research also provides insight into pitch recognition. As noted earlier, there is a close relationship in the auditory system between nerve fibers emerging from discrete areas of the basilar membrane and the pitch of the sound perceived in the brain. The fibers arising from the base of the cochlea connect with those stimulating cortical areas that perceive high pitches. Similarly, those neurons associated with the apex of the cochlea eventually stimulate the area of the brain leading to low-pitch recognition. So this orderly representation of neurons together with their variations in firing sensitivity preserve a specific relationship between place of stimulation in the cochlea, neuronal firing characteristics, physical location of final stimulation at the cortex, and pitch perception.

Over what range of frequencies is the human ear responsive? Although it extends from as low as 20 Hz to as high as 20,000 Hz (if sounds are sufficiently intense to reach auditory threshold), the frequency range over which we are *most* sensitive is considerably narrower than this. The normal ear requires the least sound pressures for tonal detection at frequencies between 500 and 4,000 Hz. This is fortunate, indeed, since this frequency range incorporates much of the power in typical human speech, particularly the less intense sounds of many high-frequency consonants so important for speech intelligibility.

Loudness

This important perceptual function seems to be associated primarily with the amount of neural energy arriving at the auditory cortex. As the intensity of our 4,000 Hz tone is increased, the stapes will continue to vibrate with the same frequency but its amplitude of movement will become greater. As a consequence, the displacement of the organ of Corti will enlarge in the area being maximally stimulated. A greater number of hair cells in that region will fire their associated neurons. Ultimately, the pitch of the stimulus will remain unchanged since the predominant neuronal grouping is maintained, but the tone will appear to be louder because the number of discharging neurons has increased.

Other Perceptual Skills

Our normal use of auditory information goes far beyond the simple designation of pitch and loudness recognition. The discrimination of human speech requires extremely fine processing skills that can differentiate complex acoustic signals varying significantly in their characteristics each fraction of a second. This task requires the auditory system to be highly functional and reasonably intact in both its peripheral and central aspects.

How do we know whether a person has normal skills in discriminating speech sounds? One way of evaluating this ability is to construct a test in which the individual is asked to identify a list of words spoken at a comfortable intensity. A test of this type is commonly used by audiologists to compare an individual's discrimination skill with that expected of persons with normal hearing. Usually a list of monosyllabic words (such as "cars," "tan," and "shoe") is presented through earphones or a loudspeaker at a comfortable loudness, and the subject is asked to repeat each word or to write it down. The *discrimination score* is determined by computing the performance of words recognized correctly. Normally hearing individuals have little difficulty in such a task if performed in quiet; their accuracy score is usually 90–100%. Because this test is so common in auditory evaluation and represents such an important communication skill, we will refer to it again from time to time when discussing auditory impairment and its effects.

Can we hear better with two ears than with one? Although the answer depends a great deal on the nature of the task, usually we are better off having the advantage of two-sided hearing. Certainly we would have great difficulty in localizing the source of sounds in our environment if we had no binaural hearing. And those with two normally functioning ears often find it easier to suppress the interference from surrounding noise when they are listening to a specific speaker. For these and other reasons, some hearing-impaired individuals find a distinct advantage to using two hearing aids rather than one.

AUDITORY REFLEXES

The auditory system plays a significant role in human life that at times is more basic than as a conduit of speech information. As we learn to associate certain sounds in our environment with aspects of danger or stress (sirens, loud shouting, etc.) or with pleasure and affection (a baby's laughter, the purring of a cat), we develop typical behavioral responses. Such actions are learned and voluntary. They depend on the central reception and processing of surrounding auditory stimuli.

Under certain conditions, however, the body may react to environmental stimuli instantaneously. Central perception may be minimal or absent. Such reactions, known as auditory reflexes, are usually mediated at subcortical levels as the auditory nervous system interacts with other motor centers in the brainstem.

Some of these reflexes are purely involuntary, representing physiologic responses of the body itself. An early example is the abrupt muscular movement of all four extremities observed as an infant is "startled" by a sharp, high-intensity sound. This response, referred to as the Moro reflex, is so common in normal infants that one might be concerned if it did not occur. Lack of such a reflex could be associated with hearing impairment, physical disabilities, or brain dysfunction.

Other involuntary reflexes to loud sound that can be observed include muscular movements around the eyes and, with special equipment, muscle reflexes in the middle ear. A typical reaction to loud, unexpected sound stimuli is blinking of the eyelids. Even a change in the dilation of the pupils may suddenly occur. Sounds of high intensity may also cause a sudden retraction of the stapedius muscle. This is called the "acoustic reflex." The tensor tympani muscle may contract in response to certain tactile stimuli. This muscular activity stiffens the ossicular chain and reduces sound flow into the cochlea. Although the reasons for such reflexes are not completely known, some believe they are meant to play a protective role.

Certain reflexes are learned and may occur without conscious intention. A good example is the combined muscular movements of the head and of the eyes as we search out the direction from which a sound of interest has emanated. Such a reaction is extremely complex. It involves binaural interaction of the two auditory inputs low in the brainstem, as previously mentioned. This information is then conveyed to the motor centers governing eye movement and the large muscle groupings of the neck and body. Although the level of sound recognition evoking such a response may be achieved at a higher neurologic level than that associated with involuntary reflexes, the listener's responses are often so immediate that conscious recognition is not involved.

IMPAIRED AUDITORY FUNCTION

The auditory system conveys information of enormous complexity to the brain, and does so with exceptionally high fidelity. This intricate mechanical and electrochemical mechanism must function well so that acoustic energy may be transmitted for appropriate processing. And in a similar way, the central nervous system with its wealth of neurologic connections must also be operational to ensure normal hearing.

We now turn our attention to the impaired auditory system. What are the implications of disorders in the conductive and/or sensorineural systems? How are such problems identified, and by whom?

The human consequences of hearing loss can be enormously varied. For some, it may be only a passing nuisance—here today, gone tomorrow. Others may adjust naturally to the effects of a slowly progressive impairment, finding it to have only a small influence in their lives. And some will have a loss of such severity, especially when occurring at an early age, that it can seriously affect their social, emotional, intellectual, and vocational potential in life.

The personal effects of reduced visual and auditory ability are often categorized into three areas. The first refers simply to reduced physiologic function—an *impairment*. Much of our discussion in this book is on this topic, demonstrating the many ways in which the ability to speak and to hear—to communicate using sound—can be compromised. The remaining two terms are concerned with the consequences of the physical impairment, potential or real. If major changes in a person's expected lifestyle ensue, a *handicap* may occur. And if the person cannot maintain gainful employment as a result of the impairment, a *disability* ensues.

> Jim has been a highly skilled metal lathe operator for over 40 years. He has been employed in a factory producing machine tools. The equipment he operates is one of a number of lathes in a large room, all of which produce such a high level of noise that Jim is unable to talk to his fellow workers. Jim is now 62. Over the past few years he has noticed that his hearing is not as good as it used to be. He has trouble hearing his wife in the next room, understanding the speaker at union meetings, and listening to the minister at church. He has constant ringing in his ears that sometimes keeps him awake at night. Of the greatest consequence, however, is the fact that he is making errors in his lathe work that have never occurred before. Jim is convinced that this happens because some of the high-frequency sounds made by his lathe during certain fashioning procedures—sounds that he has learned to rely on for accuracy in his work—are no longer perceptible to him. Jim has just received notice that his employment is to be terminated because of these errors. Jim clearly has a handicap and a disability, both consequences of an insidious auditory impairment.

HEARING EVALUATION

When an adult notices a hearing loss or develops symptoms such as ear pain or head noises, a hearing specialist is often consulted. Similarly, when a child's parents observe a lack of responsiveness to sound they will usually obtain the advice of one or more persons having specialized training in disorders of the ear and hearing. The professional services of such specialists are usually focused on one of two major areas: (1) evaluation to determine the extent, location, and cause of the problem, and (2) remediation, usually by medical, surgical, prosthetic, and/or educational means. The management of hearing loss will be considered in Chapter 9.

Hearing evaluation concerns the physical state of the ear and how well it functions. Two specialists are often involved in this activity. The physician (usually an *otologist* or *otolaryngologist*) examines the physical condition of the ear and associated structures, diagnoses the cause of the disorder, and establishes a plan of medical treatment. Determining how well the person hears is done by the *audiologist*, who may also provide nonmedical rehabilitation. These two specialists often work as a team in gathering functional and physical information so that the problem can be isolated and the most effective treatment plan devised.

Medical Examination

The physician relies on various information sources to establish a medical diagnosis and a plan for treatment. Historical information about the complaint, as described by the patient or parents, is of considerable importance. Equally helpful is knowledge of the symptoms that have been experienced. How long has the problem existed? How is it described? Did it occur suddenly or gradually over time? Is it in one or both ears? Is it associated with congenital, hereditary, infectious, or occupational factors? The answers to such questions narrow down the possible reasons for a disorder.

Although the otologist's physical examination focuses on the appearance of the ear, it certainly is not limited to that structure. The nose, mouth, and throat are carefully examined as well. Since the middle ear is directly connected to the pharynx, the condition of the respiratory tract and opening into the auditory (Eustachian) tube must be determined. The ear canal is examined while illuminating it with a bright light. Abnormal changes in the tympanic membrane (bulging, retraction, inflammation, perforation, fluid behind the drum) are often associated with middle-ear conditions. The otologist can also observe the presence of ear canal obstructions, congenital or traumatic malformations of the external ear, and visible swelling or growths due to allergies, infections, or tumors.

Since the sensorineural system is embedded within the temporal bone and central nervous system, it cannot be observed with the naked eye. However, recent developments in radiography and magnetic imaging technology provide valuable information about the physical appearance of the skull's contents. These methods, together with laboratory studies of body fluids, often provide the key that unlocks the diagnostic mystery associated with many causes of impaired hearing.

Various hearing tests can provide vital information in diagnosing ear disorders. The otologist will often use tuning forks as an efficient sound source to grossly differentiate conductive and sensorineural function. When combined with information provided by an audiologist using specialized electronic instruments, the area of dysfunction can often be localized. Once this is known, the physician narrows down the possible causes and makes a final diagnosis of the pathology involved.

Audiologic Examination

PURE-TONE AUDIOMETRY

The most widely used audiometric test is one in which a listener's minimum sensitivity (threshold) to sound is compared with that of the "average normal ear." Test equipment is calibrated so that tones of various frequencies (in Hz) can be applied at precise intensities (in dB) above those barely heard by normally hearing subjects. These physical intensity levels are defined in standards prepared by the American National Standards Institute (ANSI). The ANSI standards provide strict guidelines for checking the accuracy of equipment used throughout the country in measuring hearing. They also describe the methods used for finding audiometric thresholds.

> Since national standards define the physical properties of calibrated test equipment, the results of a specific test can be universally understood by other working health professionals. Let's suppose that the weakest 500 Hz tone just barely heard by Mrs. James in her left ear is found to be at 30 dB. All other otologists and audiologists will then know that Mrs. James requires the tone to be 30 dB more intense than the weakest tone of the same frequency that can be detected by a normal ear. We could say that Mrs. James has a hearing impairment of 30 dB above audiometric zero for that tone. If Mrs. James subsequently receives another hearing test on a different audiometer, a tone of the same physical dimensions can be easily duplicated to see whether her hearing has changed.

Tones at single, specified frequencies are presented separately under earphones at various intensities. The subject is asked to respond to each audible tone, even the faintest. In this way it is possible to determine a person's "pure-tone threshold" by finding the lowest stimulus intensity level of a tone at a specific frequency that can be detected roughly half the time it is presented. These levels can then be compared with the "normal" ANSI standards (zero decibels on the audiometer). Because the intensities used in audiometry are related to normal sensitivity, they are called *hearing levels* (HL). Thus, if Mrs. James (above) responds to about one-half the presentations of a 1,000 Hz tone at an audiometric level of 40 dB, she would be described as having a threshold of 40 dB HL.

Another designation of sound intensities used in audiometry is *sensation level* (SL). This simply refers to the number of decibels a tone is *above the threshold of a specific listener.* Thus, for Mrs. James, if the intensity dial of the audiometer is set at 50 dB HL, it would also be at 10 dB SL for that frequency (50 dB HL − 40 dB HL = 10 dB SL).

Audiometric tests are quick and reliable when the necessary equipment is in calibration and the examiner is adequately experienced and competent. The results are displayed graphically on a chart called an *audiogram.*

To examine how information is obtained for the audiogram, let us follow an audiologist through a typical test session as a cooperative adult is tested. We assume that this person has noticed a gradually progressive hearing loss in both ears for the last three years. After a hearing history and description of symptoms is obtained from the client, the ear canals are examined to ensure that they are not obstructed. The subject is then seated comfortably in a quiet environment, which is usually a sound-treated enclosure. The listener is instructed to signal by raising a hand or pushing a button immediately after each tone is heard. Earphones are carefully adjusted over each ear, and the stimulus presentations are begun in the better ear. The first threshold test is by air conduction. Remember that the sound pathway encompasses the entire auditory system (Fig. 8.3*A*). Short tone bursts are presented at a specific test frequency, with intensity varied above and below the subject's sensitivity until a threshold level is obtained. The audiologist records this level on an audiogram and then moves on to other frequencies.

The numbers across the top of the audiogram (Fig. 8.4) specify the frequencies that are typically tested in pure-tone audiometry. Although the normal human ear may be sensitive to lower and higher frequencies, those used in threshold audiometry are usually in a range between 125 and 8,000 Hz since human auditory sensitivity is most acute within these limits. In addition, the sound energy in human speech falls well within this frequency range. The numbers along the side of the audiogram (Fig. 8.4) identify the various intensity levels in decibels that are used in audiometric testing. As stated above, each level is related to the median sound pressures at which threshold responses are typically found in young, normally hearing persons. They extend from these very weak levels up to intensities as high as 110 dB above normal hearing

The 0 dB line at the top of the audiogram represents the intensity level of a calibrated audiometer at which an average normal threshold for each test frequency should occur in a quiet environment. "Normal hearing," however, is generally understood to represent hearing thresholds of less than 20 dB HL. Some hearing professionals extend the normal range up to 25 dB HL. Recent evidence indicates, however, that average sensitivity at hearing levels as low as 15–20 dB HL in the better ear may significantly affect speech and language development in some young children.

A person with a hearing impairment would, of course, require much higher sound intensities to reach a threshold. The final threshold level read by the audiologist on the intensity dial of the audiometer is transferred to the audiogram as *x* dB HL, indicating a specific intensity above audiometric zero. Various symbols are used to clarify the information on the audiogram, as shown in the box of the audiogram in Figure 8.4. Most audiologists also use red to indicate results obtained for the right ear and blue for the left.

Let us return to our hypothetical listener. The audiologist begins the test in the left ear since the listener mentioned that hearing was slightly better in that ear. It is immediately clear that the listener has impaired hearing since the tones are not heard until their levels are higher than the normal range. The air-conduction thresholds are subsequently recorded for each test frequency and for each ear.

In some cases, sensitivity may be so poor in a *unilateral* impairment that a

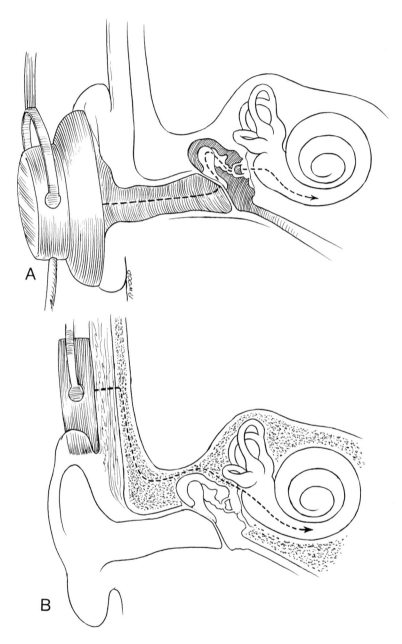

Figure 8.3.   The Air-conduction (A) and Bone-conduction (B) Pathways
Diagrams of the pathways followed by sound stimuli in air-conduction and bone-conduction audiometry.

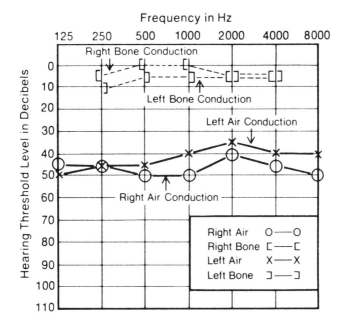

Figure 8.4. Pure-tone Audiogram of a Conductive Impairment
Hearing threshold levels found on the audiometer are depicted for each test frequency. Symbols are used to differentiate threshold levels for each ear by air and by bone conduction. This audiogram was obtained on a person with a bilateral, *conductive* hearing impairment. From Alliance of American Insurers (1981). *Technical Guide No. 9: Background for Loss of Hearing Claims,* 2nd ed. Chicago.

serious question arises about the validity of the test. Since hearing is good in the nontest ear, is it possible that the responses of the subject may be to sounds heard in the good ear? If sufficiently intense, the sound could leak from under the earphones and be heard in the opposite ear. Audiologists compensate for this problem by using a "masking" noise in the good ear while the poorer ear is retested. In this way, the good ear is busy "listening" to the nontest stimulus.

Following the completion of the air-conduction tests, the audiologist now completes the audiometric evaluation by stimulating the second pathway for sound to enter the cochlea: bone conduction (see Fig. 8.3*B*). Bone-conduction testing is carried out by presenting test tones (500 through 4,000 Hz) to a small mechanical vibrator that is attached to a headband and placed on the mastoid bone just behind the pinna of the test ear. The intensities activating the vibrator also conform to ANSI standards for bone-conduction hearing in normal ears. Our subject again signals each time the tone is sufficiently intense to reach the cochlea through the temporal bone. But which cochlea? Clearly, we are only interested in one—the mechanism on the test side. However, vibrator is closely coupled to the skull, so the entire head is being vibrated. Certainly it is possible that the normal-hearing cochlea on the left side could be responsive to the stimulus. Masking, again, is mandatory. A noise is introduced into the opposite ear through an earphone while responses are obtained from the test ear.

Our findings (Fig. 8.4) indicate depressed hearing by air conduction bilaterally. These results are perfectly consistent with the listener's history of a loss in both ears. We might say he/she has an average hearing loss by air conduction in the speech frequencies that is 40 dB HL for the left ear and 47 dB HL for the right ear. But we now know something more: we know the *type* of loss. It is due to a problem in the air-conduction pathway, *not* in the bone-conduction system. So the impairment is most likely restricted to the outer or middle ears on each side. The sensorineural system is intact.

SPEECH AUDIOMETRY

Understanding how well a person hears tones can be of considerable help in evaluating auditory function, but we cannot ignore speech as an auditory stimulus. Knowing something about the auditory processing of this more complex physical signal can provide valuable information in two dimensions. It offers cues regarding the type of impairment, and it has considerable relevance to the degree of handicap associated with the impairment. In the final analysis, the processing of tones is of significantly smaller consequence to most hearing-impaired persons than is the inability to communicate with others.

Sometimes it is helpful to compare pure-tone sensitivity with thresholds obtained for speech. This is a convenient way to check the accuracy of threshold measurements using the two different signals. The listener is asked to identify familiar words spoken at calibrated intensity levels under earphones or from a loudspeaker. Bisyllabic stimuli are used, such as "baseball," "cowboy," and "horseshoe." These words, called *spondees*, are presented in groups at hearing levels above and below threshold until one is found at which the listener can accurately repeat about half of the words spoken. This level is called a *speech reception threshold* (SRT) and is also expressed in decibels hearing level (dB HL) to indicate its relation to standardized speech sensitivity levels. The intensities at which these spondees are heard have little diagnostic significance, since they only reflect transmission through the air-conduction pathway.

A comparison of the SRT with pure-tone thresholds averaged for the audiometric frequencies in the speech range (500, 1,000, and 2,000 Hz) should be reasonably close (within ±10 dB). Discrepancies greater than this may indicate calibration problems or other factors that may need further consideration by the audiologist. The expected SRTs for the listener in Figure 8.4, for example, would be around 40 dB HL for the left ear and 50 dB HL for the right.

Another common speech test requires the listener to repeat a list of monosyllables spoken at comfortably loud levels by air conduction. This is the speech recognition test described previously. The number of words correctly identified (discrimination score) provides helpful information about the listener's ability to understand high-fidelity speech. This speech test provides insight into the degree of difficulty the listener is having in understanding the speech of others. It also offers clues as to the part of the ear involved when recognition is impaired, since those with conductive impairments perform well in this test.

OTHER TESTS

The audiologist employs a wide variety of instruments and test procedures to gather much more detailed information about auditory function when the need arises. Many of these procedures determine the listener's ability to perform a variety of behavioral tasks in response to tones and speech at various levels, both in quiet and in a background of noise. Other tests evoke physiologic responses requiring no motor behavior from the subject.

One such test, called *impedance* or *immittance audiometry,* automatically compares the acoustic energy flowing into the ear canal with the amount being reflected back from the tympanic membrane. If a disorder causes the tympanic membrane and/or ossicular chain to become stiffer than normal, more sound energy will be reflected back into the canal and be recorded by the instrument; less sound will flow through the ear than would normally be expected. These data can be of considerable importance in finding stiffness abnormalities within the mechanical system that might not otherwise be observed, thus providing valuable diagnostic information to the physician. The subject depicted in Figure 8.4 would show abnormal resistance to the flow of sound on this test.

Another procedure used by audiologists, *evoked response audiometry,* records minute electrical voltages from the auditory system as it is stimulated with certain sounds. Electrodes are attached to the head, and the tiny voltages created in the auditory system are amplified and processed by a computer. These physiologic data have important implications for how well the sensorineural system is transmitting sound into (and through) the central auditory pathways. The information gathered by this approach can provide clues regarding abnormal function in the auditory nerve and in the transmission pathways of higher neural pathways.

Sometimes, of course, the person undergoing evaluation will be rather difficult to test. This could be due to an early age, physical disabilities such as cerebral palsy, or intellectual problems. Although some of the physiologic procedures described above may be helpful, special strategies may be necessary to obtain reliable motor responses from the subject.

Jimmy was only five months old when his parents observed that he was not responding to sounds the way his older brother and sister did at this age. Their pediatrician, who did not find any obvious physical abnormality, referred Jimmy to an audiology clinic for a complete evaluation. The first tests used gross environmental stimuli (toys and noise makers) sounded behind Jimmy as he sat on his mother's lap. Jimmy was not distracted to one side or the other by these sounds, which occurred outside his field of vision. Next, the audiologist instituted a pattern of stimuli called *visual reinforcement audiometry.* With the audiologist observing Jimmy's behavior through a one-way mirror, sounds of various types and amplitudes were directed to one of two loudspeakers situated at 45° angles from Jimmy. At first, the sounds were quite loud. Immediately after each short sound presentation, a small moving toy situated next to the active speaker suddenly "came alive" for a few moments. Jimmy was delighted with this display. Soon he learned that when a sound occurred, the toy would be visible and active. In anticipation, he was conditioned to look toward the site of the active speaker if, and when, a stimulus was detected. Using this technique, Jimmy's behavioral responses to sound were found to occur at levels significantly higher than for normally hearing children of the same age. Results of evoked response audiometry also indicated that Jimmy's auditory nervous system was severely impaired. Although further tests would be conducted as Jimmy matured, it was clear to the audiologist that an effective auditory habilitation plan should be instituted for Jimmy immediately.

SYMPTOMS AND CAUSES

There are many ways to group the various etiologies responsible for impaired hearing. The plan used here will describe the various symptoms and causes that are primarily associated with the functional parts of the ear covered earlier in this chapter. We begin with impairments of the conductive mechanism, then discuss those of the sensorineural and central perceptive systems.

Conductive Impairments

In the earlier discussion of normal auditory function, the ear was separated into two major divisions in order to reflect the very different transmission modes of each. It is equally appropriate to do the same when considering the auditory system in its abnormal state. A conductive impairment refers to a reduction in auditory function associated with a disorder in the mechanical or acoustic pathway. The problem may involve the outer or middle ear or both. The delicate cochlear end organ and associated neurons carrying stimuli to the brain are intact and completely functional.

SYMPTOMS

A conductive impairment occurs because sound energy flowing through the outer and/or middle ear is impeded. The individual's sensitivity for surrounding sound is therefore reduced, but hearing by bone conduction is significantly better than by air conduction.

Hearing-impaired individuals often complain of two problems in addition to a sensitivity loss. The first is associated with speech perception and the second with noises within the ear or the head that appear to have no relation to surrounding auditory stimuli (*tinnitus*). Although persons with a bilateral conductive loss may wish others to speak louder in order to surmount their sensitivity loss, they do *not* complain of difficulty in speech understanding. Since their sensorineural mechanism is functional, speech intelligibility is normal as long as it is at a comfortable level above speech threshold. Tinnitus is often described as buzzing, hissing, or ringing sensations that are especially loud in quiet settings. Although most commonly associated with sensorineural conditions, tinnitus does occur in some conductive impairments as well. The etiology of continuous tinnitus is not fully understood, but it can be associated with many causes of impaired hearing.

So, those with a conductive impairment typically have one major auditory complaint: a loss of sensitivity. It may occur in one or both ears and within a wide range of severity. It can never cause a total impairment, however, since the sensorineural system is still intact. Tinnitus may or may not be present.

CAUSES

How do these conductive impairments occur? What etiologic factors are responsible? Let us examine the more common of them.

Obstructed Ear Canal

A complete blockage of the ear canal would clearly result in a significant reduction in auditory sensitivity. A partial obstruction should not produce a major impairment, but might make the canal diameter so small that closure could easily occur intermittently in the presence of excess moisture or ear wax (*cerumen*). Since the shape and circumference of the ear canal vary widely from person to person, some individuals may notice such problems more than others.

Obstructed ear canals are usually due to one of the following: cerumen accumulation in the canal; some foreign object inserted into the canal; malformations of the canal during fetal development; and abnormal growths occurring on the canal wall. The presence of these abnormalities can be observed readily during a physical examination of the ears.

Dysfunction of the Middle-Ear Transformer

Conditions preventing the normal process of converting acoustic to mechanical energy and then transmitting it into the cochlear fluids will clearly lead to serious impairments in auditory function. Normal sensitivity demands that the sound energy arriving unobstructed at the tympanic membrane be conveyed to the cochlear end organ in the most efficient manner possible. A number of problems might disrupt the normal movement of the transformer mechanism.

A common cause of conductive impairments is *middle-ear infection,* often due to *auditory (Eustachian) tube dysfunction.* As mentioned before, normal tube function is critical in providing pressure equalization between the surrounding air and that in the middle-ear cavity. Periodic openings of the auditory tube maintain this normal balance. If the tube stays closed for a prolonged period, however, the air trapped in the cavity is slowly absorbed by the cells lining its walls. This causes a vacuum to be formed in this space as the air pressure becomes less and less. The greater atmospheric pressure in the ear canal pushes the tympanic membrane into the cavity, stretching and stiffening the membrane. Its ability to respond to the minute periodic changes in air pressure exerted by weak sounds is reduced, and a hearing loss occurs. Impaired hearing would also ensue if the pressure inside the middle ear were *greater* than that in the environment and it could not be voluntarily equalized by opening the auditory tube. These conditions are sometimes experienced during or after air travel, when the auditory tube's normal function is impeded by a cold or an allergic reaction. Scuba divers can also experience this problem if they are unable to adjust for the necessary pressure changes in their environment. If negative pressure remains in the middle ear for a day or two, the resulting vacuum may draw a clear fluid from the cells lining the middle-ear cavity. This fluid is called *effusion*. As it begins to accumulate in the ear, its presence contributes further to the conductive loss.

If bacteria enter the middle ear, a full-blown infection could easily result. This is particularly common in children. Inflammation and pain develop, the effusion becomes thick and yellow, and the tympanic membrane is affected by pressure changes and tissue swelling. Certainly a hearing loss will be present, although the concurrent pain, fever, and discomfort generally take precedence among the symptoms.

If this condition is not properly treated, usually with antibiotic drugs, the infectious process can spread to other structures and cause serious damage. It can invade the mastoid process of the temporal bone, just behind the pinna. It can break down the tissue of the tympanic membrane in a particular spot, causing a sudden perforation. If this should occur, the pus in the middle ear would now have an escape avenue (a "draining" ear) and the pain of the infection might be reduced, but the underlying cause would remain. In some cases, individuals have had such chronic conditions for years. The continuing infectious process may attack important structures, such as the ossicles and surrounding bone. If the infection breaks down the wall separating the middle ear and the brain cavity, the brain lining can become involved (meningitis). Even after a bacterial infection of the middle ear is successfully treated, any resultant scarring, adhesions, and tympanic perforation can continue to impede the transformer function so important to normal sensitivity.

All of the conditions described above are generically referred to as *otitis media*. When accompanied by infection, especially of a chronic nature as just discussed, the problem may have serious implications for general health.

Abnormal function of the auditory tube can also result from allergic reactions associated with generalized swelling of tissue in the throat, a condition not unlike that occurring in the early stages of a cold.

A person born with a cleft of the hard or soft palate often has periodic infections of the middle ear because the muscular control of the auditory tube opening is abnormal. Improper development of these muscles prevents normal tube operation, and hearing loss is almost inevitable.

Another obstructive condition of the middle ear is *otosclerosis*. This is an abnormal growth of bony tissue at the base of the stapes in the oval window. As this condition slowly enlarges, the motion of the stapes footplate within the window is gradually reduced and hearing sensitivity decreases accordingly. This is not a cancerous condition, and there is no pain. Although the cause is not certain, there seems to be a significant hereditary factor in some cases. It may occur in one ear only, but is often a bilateral condition.

In addition to *genetic malformations* of the outer or middle ears that are present at birth, structural deviations may occur later in life. These may occur because of growths in the middle ear or as a result of physical injuries to the transformer mechanism. Examples include the force of sudden air pressures into the canal (an explosion, slap to the ear, or insertion of something into the canal) or blows against the head resulting in skull fractures or a disarticulation of the ossicles. Any conditions of this nature resulting in depressed mechanical function will lead to a conductive impairment as long as the sensorineural system remains normal.

MEDICAL FINDINGS

Fortunately, most of the modalities described above can be observed directly through the ear canal. Pressure changes in the middle ear, infections, and the presence of effusion typically lead to an abnormal-appearing tympanic membrane. Physical trauma is equally obvious when it involves the membrane. In some conditions, however, the physician may need to perform exploratory surgery to confirm the diagnosis. Lifting the tympanic membrane to peer into the middle ear cavity will usually confirm the presence of otosclerosis, an ossicular disarticulation, or a tumor. Infections are sometimes revealed by an elevated body temperature and laboratory studies of body fluids. Since the site of the abnormality is often visible, it can usually be treated successfully by drugs and/or surgical intervention.

AUDIOLOGIC FINDINGS

Pure-tone audiometry typically shows depressed thresholds for air-conducted stimuli (see Fig. 8.4). Bone-conduction sensitivity will be normal. Often all frequencies are affected, showing a flat loss, but the low frequencies can be more depressed than the highs. Speech discrimination scores will be in the normal range (90–100%) since the speech intensity is raised to compensate for the sensitivity loss and no problem exists in the sensorineural system. Abnormal findings on immittance audiometry are very common, reflecting changes in sound flow associated with dysfunction of the mechanical transformer.

Ruth is a 32-year-old secretary whose hearing had been normal until she was 30. She remembered that her grandmother had developed a hearing loss in later life, but had assumed it was associated with her age. Ruth's hearing seemed to become worse gradually, and about equally in both ears. Her own voice seemed to be quite loud to her, although others complained that she "didn't talk as loudly" as she used to. She reported no noises in her head, dizziness, or aural pain.

Her physician sent her to an otologist for a thorough evaluation. No physical abnormalities were found in her ears or respiratory tract. Auditory tests indicated that she heard much better by bone conduction than by air conduction in each ear. Her audiogram was similar to that depicted in Figure 8.4. Her ability to understand speech, when sufficiently amplified to overcome her sensitivity loss, was completely unimpaired. The otologist tentatively diagnosed her conductive loss as due to otosclerosis in the absence of any physical signs. This diagnosis was confirmed during subsequent surgery on Ruth's right ear. After cutting the skin around the tympanic membrane and moving it aside temporarily, the otologist used a powerful microscope to observe the abnormal tissue growth at the stapes footplate. (The surgical procedure used to correct this condition, called *stapedectomy,* is described in Chapter 9.)

Sensorineural Impairments

Impaired function of the sensorineural system includes any condition affecting the normal operation of the sensory end organ, of the associated neural pathways to the brain, and/or of the auditory cortex itself. Problems occur either in the complex transduction of sound energy into neural stimulation in the cochlea or in the transmission and perception capability of the auditory nervous system. In either event, the physical characteristics of sound entering the cochlea by air or bone conduction are not accurately transmitted or centrally coded by the brain. Sound cues related to frequency, intensity, and time are not faithfully reproduced at the auditory cortex, often resulting in a distortion of the sound stimulus *in addition* to a sensitivity loss.

SYMPTOMS

Disorders of the sensorineural system can result in wide degrees of hearing loss and can occur in one or both ears simultaneously. The same is true of conductive impairments. But there the similarity ends. It is possible that a profound loss may occur, for example—one considerably greater than that possible in a conductive problem. Tinnitus is commonly experienced, either intermittently or continuously, and of varied intensity and quality.

One of the major complaints distinguishing conductive and sensorineural disorders relates to speech intelligibility. Those with sensorineural impairments often find it difficult to understand the speech of others, even though it is sufficiently loud to overcome whatever sensitivity loss may occur. The problem is compounded in listening environments that are noisy, or when groups of people are speaking at once.

> Mr. Roman, now 68 years old, had begun to notice a hearing loss four years previously. It was very mild at first—instances when he noticed that he did not hear birds sing as well as he had or missed the ring of a telephone that was obviously heard by others. As time went on, these absences of sound became accentuated. But in addition, he began having problems understanding the speech of others even though they seemed to be talking at a normal loudness. The problem was worse at parties or when talking to his wife on the bus. He also noticed that a continuous, high-pitched tone was present in both ears when he went to bed at night.

CAUSES

The etiologic factors responsible for sensorineural losses can be considered in relation to the structures responsible for two major functions in the sensorineural system: (1) transduction of mechanical to electrical energy in the cochlea, and (2) transmission and perception of stimuli in the neural pathways.

Dysfunction of the Hair-Cell Transducer

Impaired hearing associated with the aging process is commonly referred to as *presbycusis*. It should be of little surprise that Mr. Roman's problem in the above illustration is due to this condition. Certain membranes and tissues within the body are known to develop a restricted range of motion with aging, becoming stiffer than normal. Should this happen to the movable cochlear membranes, the energy transfer within the cochlear partition could be reduced with subsequent lack of hair-cell stimulation and neural transmission. Such a condition is not necessarily present in all those with hearing impairments due to aging, but it can be a contributing factor in some cases. Usually impaired hearing due to aging is a bilateral occurrence, producing similar degrees of impairment in each ear. Presbycusis may be due to factors other than structural stiffness, however. These might include cellular deterioration of the organ of Corti itself and changes in cell chemistry that might prevent normal firing of the end organ.

A distinctive instigator of hearing impairment associated with hair-cell dysfunction is a condition called *Meniere's* (pronounced "men yairz'") disease. The major symptoms are a sudden occurrence of severe dizziness and nausea (vertigo) accompanied by a hearing loss and tinnitus. It is usually confined to one ear, although bilateral conditions do occur. Needless to say, the vertigo is usually the symptom of greatest concern at the onset of the disorder. It is often so severe that the individual is unable to walk normally until the attack recedes, usually within a few hours. The hearing loss and tinnitus usually remain, although they may become less severe over time. Unfortunately, repeated attacks of the symptoms may occur without warning in some individuals. The cause of Meniere's disease is not fully understood. It does seem to be associated, however, with the production of excessive endolymphatic fluid in the cochlea and connecting labyrinth.

> Ms. Crandle had never had problems with her hearing until that day in June a few years ago. As she was walking down the street after shopping, she suddenly became so disoriented that she fell down. The "dizzy spell" became so intense that she was unable to gain her feet. In addition, she became quite nauseous, vomiting where she lay. Clearly, she was physically and emotionally distressed. Soon it also became clear that her hearing in one ear was quite poor, and a low-pitched roaring noise was constant in that ear. The dizziness experienced by Ms. Crandle gradually disappeared within an hour, but the hearing loss and tinnitus remained. She experienced four more episodes of these dizzy spells over the next three years, with fluctuating hearing and tinnitus over the same period.

In addition to structural changes affecting mechanical stimulation of the hair cells, the cells themselves could be compromised by additional factors leading to dysfunction of normal energy transfer in specific areas of the cochlea or along most of the basilar membrane. Various causes might be implicated.

Developmental malformations can involve the inner ear as well as the outer and middle ears. Arrested or abnormal growth of the temporal bone space and contents can result from genetic abnormalities or toxicity accompanying maternal infection or drug ingestion. Normally such conditions show their effects early in embryonic development, since the cochlear structure is almost completely formed by the end of the first three months after conception.

Trauma to the organ of Corti may result from external blows to the skull leading to fractures through the cochlea. Such accidents may cause sudden breaks or tears in the bony walls of the cochlea, in the cochlear membranes, in the organ of Corti, or in the peripheral nervous system. Such trauma usually occurs quite suddenly and is often on only one side, and the resultant change in audition is noticed immediately. These events are quite rare, however, compared with the physical damage to the hair cells that can occur as a result of noise exposure.

Noise-induced impairments usually develop over a prolonged period. As certain hair cells are bombarded with high levels of sound, their function begins to change. A temporary hearing loss accompanied by ringing tinnitus is not unusual after certain exposure periods, indicating a physical change in normal hair-cell function. Repeated exposure to sound levels causing these symptoms can be cumulative in its effect. Permanent sensitivity shifts begin to occur in the higher frequencies, spreading into lower frequencies with continued exposure. So the initial physical damage caused by high noise levels begins toward the base of the cochlea.

Hearing impairment due to noise is becoming common in our highly complex (and increasingly noisy) society. It has been noted primarily in adults in the past, and has been more common in men than women. This reflected greater exposure of men over 21 to industrial noise, gun fire, etc. However, in recent years evidence has been mounting of permanent impairments in women who have been exposed to industrial noise. Similarly, significant changes have been observed in younger people of college age. Some experts believe this is sometimes associated with music listening habits that have become popular in the last 20 years. Generally, permanent damage due to noise requires exposure periods that are relatively long, unless the noise is unusually intense or occurs as a sharp wave front (such as in a blast or explosion). The effects are somewhat variable, however. Some individuals seem to have "tougher" ears than others, and a small percentage appear to be unusually susceptible to such exposures.

A complicating factor in determining whether a sensorineural impairment is due solely to noise, however, is the association of such impairments with various *degenerative* problems in later life. Changes in the structural integrity of the hair cells and associated membranes have already been referred to. Such effects may be related to generalized changes associated with aging, or they could be the result of obscure hereditary abnormalities that develop in adulthood.

Certain conditions affecting the normal chemical balance within and external to the hair cells will disrupt the ability of the cell to stimulate associated neurons. Such *metabolic* abnormalities may be associated with diabetes, hypoglycemia, and hypothyroidism, and the consequences of protein (Rh) incompatibility between the parents of newborn children. Unless the chemical environment surrounding the hair cells is suitable and proper nutrients are present in the cochlear fluids, the transduction process so necessary to neural stimulation can be compromised.

Vascular disorders can also interrupt the normal status of hair cells by obstructing the flow of oxygen to the cochlea. This might occur as a result of an occlusion in a blood vessel or a sudden break in the vessel wall. Such vascular accidents may be associated with arteriosclerosis, high blood pressure, and similar conditions. Disorders of this type are often responsible for sudden hearing impairments that seem to have no obvious cause.

A wide variety of *infectious processes* can be responsible for reduced hair-cell function. Bacteria from middle-ear infections can invade the cochlea through a breakdown of the membranes or bone separating the two parts of the ear. They may also attack the cochlear end organ as agents of a specific disease, such as syphilis. A variety of viruses are also responsible for sensory disorders. Those that are particularly relevant are associated with rubella (German measles), mumps, regular measles, and some forms of influenza.

Finally, the delicate structure of the cochlear end organ is susceptible to damage from various *ototoxic* agents that may find their way into the system. Some powerful antibiotic drugs are particularly known for their ototoxic potential, as are certain diuretic agents. Again, as in the case of noise as an etiologic factor, variations in individual susceptibility to the toxic effects of such drugs have been observed.

Disrupted Neurologic Transmission and Perception

Many of the conditions described above may also impair auditory nerve function, reduce transmission within the central nervous system, or affect the normal auditory perception occurring in the brain. *Degenerative changes* in the neural structures can occur throughout the system. They can develop quite slowly in association with aging or *tumors* developing at the floor of the skull, brainstem, or cortex. Bacterial or viral *infections* may involve neural tissue directly or may cause damage as a consequence of high fevers accompanying some of these diseases. Disorders causing *metabolic changes* in the nervous system include those that may affect hair-cell function mentioned above (except Meniere's disease). An additional disease, specific to the nervous system, is *multiple sclerosis*. This condition breaks down the insulating myelin sheath of the nerve, thereby impairing neural functioning. Fortunately, periods of remission are characteristic, and hearing may improve for certain periods.

Traumatic injury to the skull from external forces can also damage neural and/ or brain tissue. Prenatal lack of oxygen or *hypoxia* during birth or following vascular accidents within the skull may also result in physical damage to the auditory nervous system. As noted in Chapter 5, vascular disorders such as occlusions or sudden breaks in vessel walls can have a devastating effect on communicative functioning if they occur in the dominant hemisphere for speech and/or hearing (usually in the left temporal lobe). Strokes in this area may lead to auditory aphasia, a condition in which the listener's sensitivity to speech may be intact but speech understanding is poor.

MEDICAL FINDINGS

Since the sensorineural system is not readily observable, the physician must rely on information from various sources to evaluate auditory dysfunction and diagnose the cause. The radiographic and imaging techniques referred to earlier can be of considerable assistance in determining the presence of neoplastic growths within the skull or the unusual positioning of soft tissues in response to abnormal fluid or tumor pressure. Similarly, traumatic injuries can often be observed with such techniques. Laboratory studies, including examination of the normally clear spinal fluid, can indicate abnormal bleeding, excessive fluid pressure within the system, and the presence of infection.

Since many of the cranial nerves are located in close proximity to the auditory nerve, the physician carefully explores the function of each. In addition to the information obtained by the audiologist regarding the auditory system, careful attention is also given to the operation of the balance mechanism. Disorders affecting either the cochlea or the auditory nerve may also involve elements of the sensory vestibular mechanism and associated aspects of cranial nerve VIII. After stimulating the vestibular system, abnormal function can be detected by observing and electrically recording muscular activity around the eyes (*electronystagmography*). Since there is a close connection in the brainstem between the vestibular and ocular systems, sudden stimulation of a single vestibular end organ normally produces involuntary movements of the eyes for a short period (nystagmus). The configuration and strength of these movements (or the lack thereof) can offer valuable clues in auditory diagnosis.

AUDIOLOGIC FINDINGS

Although the average pure-tone threshold may be quite variable in sensorineural impairments, certain characteristics are commonly seen. Sensitivity, of course, will be similar whether determined using the air- or bone-conduction pathways. And since presbycusis is the most common etiologic factor in such impairments, the typical audiogram of the older adult will show *better sensitivity in the low frequencies than in the high frequencies* (Fig. 8.5). Such an audiogram might be seen in a person such as Mr. Roman (see above). The configuration may be quite variable, however, depending on the underlying cause.

A major distinction of sensorineural impairments, compared with conductive system impairments, is observed when evaluating speech recognition ability. Although a wide range of discrimination scores may occur, they are typically depressed. Individuals with cochlear impairments often have discrimination scores as low as 40% or 50%. Many with disorders of the auditory nerve may show scores considerably poorer than this. Such problems reflect the system's inability to adequately transduce physical energy at the hair-cell level or transmit it through a restricted population of nerve fibers in the auditory nerve. Because the number of fibers increase dramatically once the brainstem is reached, individuals with abnormalities of the central nervous system may not demonstrate problems in hearing pure-tone and undistorted speech. These stimuli are not sufficiently complex to require maximum neurologic activity in their perception. The audiologist must therefore use highly distorted speech to detect abnormal functioning within the central system, including the auditory cortex. Such stimuli may include speech combined with noise, speeded speech, speech with high frequencies removed, etc.

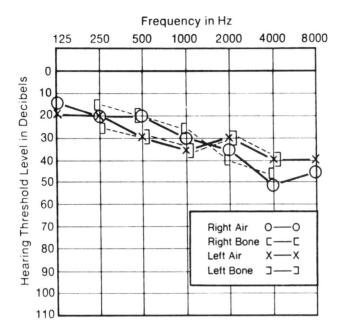

Figure 8.5. Pure-tone Audiogram of a Sensorineural Impairment
Air- and bone-conduction audiograms of a person with a bilateral, *sensorineural* impairment. Note that there is no "gap" in sensitivity between the air and bone thresholds for either ear. From Alliance of American Insurers (1981). *Technical Guide No. 9: Background For Loss of Hearing Claims*, 2nd ed. Chicago.

John, aged 36, had never had a problem with his hearing until he first noticed eight months ago that sound sensitivity in his left ear was worse than in his right. Since then, his hearing loss has progressed and sound quality seems to be distorted. He notices a high-pitched, ringing noise in the left ear, especially when it is quiet. He has also had periodic headaches in the last year and experiences some "dizziness" from time to time.

Otologic and audiologic examination revealed reduced vestibular function on the left and confirmed his hearing loss. Sensitivity was equally depressed for air and bone conduction in the left ear. Discrimination of speech spoken at a comfortably loud level was very poor in the left ear; John could understand only six of 50 monosyllables spoken in that ear. The otologist recommended radiographic and magnetic resonance imaging studies of John's skull. These tests revealed definite evidence of a small growth that could be impinging on cranial nerve VIII, causing both auditory and vestibular dysfunction. John was then referred to a neurosurgeon for further evaluation and to help determine whether surgery should be undertaken to remove the tumor.

We have seen, then, that the person with sensorineural impairment may be burdened not only with a loss in sensitivity, but also with difficulty in discriminating among many of the phonemes in speech. Because of damage to the analysis system in the cochlea or to the transmission capacity of the auditory nerve (or to both), the spectral characteristics of many speech sounds are missing or distorted by the time they reach the cortical perception centers.

Unfortunately, a third auditory problem is often associated with sensorineural impairments. Certain individuals find their *tolerance* for loud sounds is decreased. This symptom is most predominant in those with cochlear pathology. Even though the person's threshold is elevated, the high-intensity levels causing discomfort may remain constant or even become lower. Consequently, the decibel range over which the ear is able to operate (from sensitivity threshold to discomforting loudness) is restricted compared with the normal ear. Such a person may thus have difficulty adjusting to hearing aids unless they are built to amplify only within the listener's operating range.

As mentioned earlier, the audiologist may use special tests to help determine the locus of the disorder within this complex system. Such tests may evaluate special aspects of auditory behavior known to be involved in disorders of the cochlea, the nerve, or the central pathways and cortex. They may reflect the ability of the listener to balance the loudness of tones between the ears or to maintain sensitivity to continuous presentation of weak sounds over time. Such behavioral tests are often supplemented by more objective techniques designed to evoke electrical activity within the auditory system. Certain disorders often cause quite abnormal responses that can be of considerable value in auditory diagnosis.

Nonorganic Problems

From time to time, persons are identified who appear to have a significant hearing impairment but have little or no physiologic basis for their behavior. Usually such individuals consciously "depress" their hearing sensitivity in an attempt to reap a monetary reward or perhaps to obtain special attention to satisfy an emotional need. In rare instances, such behavior might be on an unconscious basis, resulting from severe psychologic trauma. Whatever the cause, such conditions are referred to as a "functional" hearing problem or, more recently, as *pseudohypacusis*. Generally, those who consciously feign a hearing impairment find it difficult to maintain consistent behavioral responses to auditory tests performed by audiologists and otologists, and many of the physiologically based procedures discussed above will indicate better sensitivity than that admitted by the individual. Pseudohypacusis on an unconscious basis, however, most usually will be diagnosed by a psychiatrist.

SUMMARY

This chapter has explored the physical dimensions of a system that provides the unique links between the acoustic emissions of the human speaker and the linguistic capabilities of the human listener. Acoustic energy entering the outer ear is transmitted by the mechanical action of the middle ear into hydrodynamic activity within the cochlea of the inner ear. Stimulation of the hair cells initiates neurologic transmission of the signal, leading to central processing within the brain.

Figure 8.6 summarizes the major causes of hearing impairment relative to the site that is most often involved in each condition. But it does something more: it provides

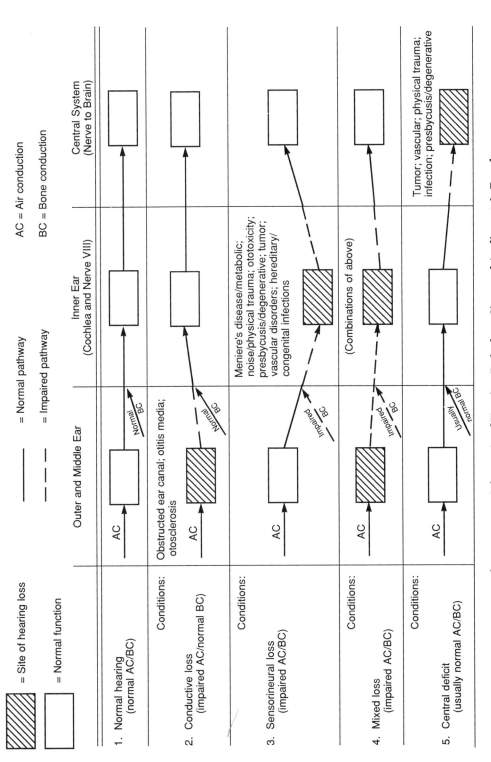

Figure 8.6. Summary Schematic of Hearing Pathology Sites and Audiometric Results

Hearing impairments, their sites in the auditory system, the primary pathologies associated with each site, and expected results obtained with pure-tone audiometry. Central deficits are often called sensorineural impairments, especially when associated with reduced sensitivity to tones.

information on the type of impaired function that can be observed in pure-tone audiometry. The category entitled "mixed loss" has not been specifically addressed above; it simply represents the presence of a conductive and a sensorineural impairment together. Such impairments often result from more than one pathology, but in some instances could be due to a single cause. An example would be a person with severe otosclerosis in which the abnormal growth around the oval window causes secondary destruction within the cochlea. The category labeled "central deficit" relates to impaired function in the central nervous system. We discussed these problems as occurring in the sensorineural system, but emphasized that they usually do not include reduced sensitivity to tones. This is because the central system is so "rich" with neural units that even when impaired it can still perform the comparatively simple task of recognizing a tone close to threshold. Very few nerve elements are necessary for this function.

SUGGESTED READINGS

The following two texts cover the physical aspects of sound as an acoustic signal, a description of the ear's structure and function, and how sound is normally perceived. They are excellent introductions to more detailed information on each of these topics. Additional references are provided for serious students of human audition.

Durrant, J. D. and J. H. Lovrinic, (1984). *Bases of Hearing Science,* 2nd ed. Baltimore: Williams & Wilkins.
Yost, W. A., and D. W. Nielsen, (1985). *Fundamentals of Hearing: An Introduction,* 2nd ed. New York: Holt, Rinehart & Winston.

These two English authors discuss their topics in somewhat more detail than is given in the previous books, but in highly readable formats.

Moore, B. C. J. (1982). *An Introduction to the Psychology of Hearing,* 2nd ed. New York: Academic Press. *This text covers perceptive aspects of loudness, pitch, auditory patterning, and speech perception.*
Pickles, J. O. (1982). *An Introduction to the Physiology of Hearing.* New York: Academic Press. *The focus is on auditory physiology, with special attention to the inner ear and auditory nervous system.*

The following three textbooks are popular introductions to the field of audiology. They comprise material relevant to all aspects of hearing and its disorders. Each of them covers auditory disorders and provides substantive information on basic audiometric tests using tones and speech.

Davis, H., and S. R. Silverman, (1978). *Hearing and Deafness,* 4th ed. New York: Holt, Rinehart & Winston.
Martin, F. N. (1986). *Introduction to Audiology,* 3rd ed. Englewood Cliffs, NJ: Prentice-Hall.
Newby, H., and G. R. Popelka, (1985). *Audiology,* 5th ed. Englewood Cliffs, NJ: Prentice-Hall.

A more advanced treatment of audiology is found in the following:

Martin, F. N. (Ed.) (1981). *Medical Audiology: Disorders of Hearing.* Englewood Cliffs, NJ: Prentice-Hall. *This text takes the reader through the divisions of the ear (outer and inner ears, cochlea, auditory nerve, and central system). In addition to anatomic and physiologic considerations, each section covers pertinent aspects of pathology, audiology/otologic diagnosis, and management. Excellent examples are given of how information provided by the two disciplines of otology and audiology is melded into professional decisions regarding hearing impairment.*

Those who are seeking detailed information on auditory pathology and otologic treatment should, of course, consult recent textbooks in otology that can be found in any medical library. We particularly recommend the following:

Schuknecht, H. F. (1974). *Pathology of the Ear.* Cambridge, MA: Harvard University Press. *A classic in providing exceptional reviews of aural diseases and their treatment. References to the literature are exhaustive, and graphic illustrations are excellent.*

Study Questions

1. Imagine the movements of the prongs of a tuning fork once it is hit against something and produces a sound. Describe how these movements relate to the pitch and loudness of the fork as you hear it.

2. Using the same concept as above, think in terms of what is happening to the ear as the sound from the tuning fork passes through the ear to the brain. What do the eardrum and ossicles do in response to the sound waves that hit it? How are the fluids of the cochlea placed into motion? How are the intensity and frequency of the fork's motions conveyed so accurately into the auditory nerve?

3. What do you suppose might happen to the operation of the ear if there were a hole in the eardrum? Do you think things would be better or worse if somehow a separation occurred in the connection of the incus with the stapes? Why?

4. Imagine that an individual has a hearing loss in the high frequencies, say above 1,000 Hz. What types of speech sounds might be hard for that person to hear?

5. An individual who normally has good hearing wakes up one morning with one ear canal completely plugged with wax. In the shower, he/she notices hearing the sound of water hitting the head and back, and that it appears to be loudest in the left ear. Which ear is plugged? How did you arrive at this conclusion?

6. Refer to the first clinical illustration. List the potential handicapping circumstances in Jim's life as a result of his impairment. In what way may his speech articulation be different than it was before the onset of his impairment?

7. Why might one find more valid and reliable evidence about a person's hearing sensitivity using an audiometer rather than a tuning fork?

8. Which do you think would be a more accurate measure of auditory sensitivity: air conduction or bone conduction? Why?

9. Why do you suppose a person with a stroke that has affected the auditory area of the left hemisphere is unable to understand the speech of others, but still has a relatively normal pure-tone audiogram?

9

Managing Hearing Impairment

How can hearing be restored? What can be done if the impairment is permanent? Answers to these questions, when applied to the needs of specific individuals, will vary depending upon a number of factors influencing the current status of the hearing problem. These factors may play a significant role in the future impact of the impairment. They include, among others, the physical cause of the problem, the age at onset, the degree of severity, its consistency over time, the part of the ear affected, the person's age, and the influence of the impairment on the individual's past and present life (social, emotional, vocational, and educational). Many of these matters were discussed in Chapter 8 as potential consequences of auditory dysfunction, but they vary so extensively from one person to the next that they must be carefully evaluated in each case. Hearing impairment can often be reversed, and the implications of permanent conditions can be addressed in positive ways. We will explore strategies for doing so in this chapter. But first we consider some implications of impaired hearing. Since one is immediately confronted with a list of descriptors when discussing this issue, we begin by reviewing some applicable terminology.

LABELING THE HEARING PROBLEM

Abnormal function may be described in many ways. The following words are commonly applied to hearing: hearing loss, hearing impairment, hard-of-hearing, the hearing impaired, the deaf, and deafness. Do these terms all apply to the same thing? Some with limited knowledge of the problem may think that they do. Others may assume that all persons having any difficulty with their hearing are "deaf." Persons who are impaired often use clear distinctions when interpreting the meaning of these words, and these interpretations often differ from those used by others.

The descriptors just referred to are most often used in the same context: to describe a person or condition associated with "abnormal" hearing. Hearing professionals and those with severe impairments often select from among these descriptors according to a more subtle designation of *degree* or *severity*—as we shall do here. The words "deaf" or "deafness" usually connote a more severe degree of functional loss than do the other terms. But in what context is "severity" defined? Is it simply a person's sensitivity to sound compared with that of a "normally hearing" person?

We could differentiate the degree of impaired function solely on the basis of audiometric threshold criteria. Indeed, such an approach is widely used as a convenient way to describe the *level* of hearing impairment. A person having an average pure-tone threshold at a hearing level of 30 dB in the better ear would have less of an impairment, in this context, than a person with a 60 dB HL threshold. A table of popular modifiers has been developed to describe this relation between average pure-tone air-conduction threshold and severity of impairment (Table 9.1). Hearing impairments in each ear can be classified from "mild" to "profound" with such descriptors, and often are so designated for a variety of purposes.

Although such methods are not completely standardized as to hearing levels, they are often used as general ways to provide comparative information about impairment. They represent varied levels of difficulty often experienced by the hearing impaired when listening to the conversational speech of others. Such a classification is highly simplistic, however, and is a grossly inadequate means of differentiating the hearing impaired according to their comparative communicative skills. A person's ability to utilize effectively whatever residual audition remains depends on many factors in addition to sensitivity for tones. For example, the designators in Table 9.1 refer to *monaural* impairment. The application of this scale to the total auditory capacity of a listener would clearly need to consider hearing in the other ear. It cannot be used to describe the handicapping degree of a hearing loss.

The primary distinction between a hard-of-hearing person and a deaf person is generally based on how well remaining auditory function in both ears is used in interhuman speech communication. The *deaf* person finds little practical help from residual hearing, usually because auditory function is insufficient to adequately recognize the speech of others by audition alone. The visual channel becomes the primary

Table 9.1.   Scale of Hearing Impairment

AVERAGE THRESHOLD LEVEL (dB HL)[a]	SUGGESTED DESCRIPTION[b]
0–15	Normal hearing
16–25	Slight hearing loss
26–40	Mild hearing loss
41–55	Moderate hearing loss
56–70	Moderately severe hearing loss
71–90	Severe hearing loss
91 plus	Profound hearing loss

[a] Decibels are referenced to average normal hearing for 500, 1,000, and 2,000 Hz under earphones.
[b] These descriptors are used primarily for unilateral impairment.

means of receiving ideas and information from others, with supplementation by audition to the degree that it is available. Even when a hearing aid is employed, speech understanding through the auditory pathway is often so poor that primary reliance must be placed on visual recognition skills. The use of manual-coded sign systems to depict objects, concepts, and individual letters of the alphabet is the predominant mode of communication, supplemented by "reading" the lips and the facial and body movements of the speaker.

The *hard-of-hearing* person, on the other hand, is able to use auditory sensations effectively and therefore relies on the ears as the predominant perceptive mode. These individuals may receive substantial assistance from hearing aids. Enhanced visual skills strongly supplement the sensory input of the listener. But spoken language is normally the primary means of conveying ideas to others.

CONSEQUENCES OF HEARING IMPAIRMENT

Our discussion of impaired hearing thus far has focused almost exclusively on reduced hearing for tones and speech. Clearly, such problems represent the most obvious result of hearing dysfunction. But a loss of audition may lead to consequences that go considerably beyond the communicative impairment itself. Recent studies indicate that about 13 million Americans have a significant reduction in hearing efficiency. For many of these people, additional factors attributable to their impairment also govern their lives. Differences in the personal behavior of the hearing impaired are associated with variables that can have a profound influence on how persons cope with their impairment. These include not only the degree and type of hearing loss, as described above, but the age of onset and of intervention and the response of the person to amplification and special education, which will be of great importance in the degree of handicap or disability.

Jenny and Bill were both born in 1964. Although they were apparently robust and physically normal at birth, Bill was soon found to be completely unresponsive to environmental sound. Jenny's auditory responsiveness was typical of a normally hearing child. Jenny spent her early childhood in a sound-rich environment, learning language and speech skills without hindrance. She was speaking in sentences by age three, was reading simple primers at five, and was writing single words at six. Bill, whose parents were deaf, had no oral speech at the age of six. He had already learned to communicate effectively with his parents and their friends using manual signs, however. Because of the severity of his sensorineural loss and his parent's past experiences, he did not wear hearing aids.

At the age of six, Jenny contracted mumps. Within a few days her hearing was gone. Both she and Bill had similarly profound impairments. Powerful hearing aids were provided for Jenny at each ear. These provided vibratory stimulation to her ear canals that may have been useful to her in giving her sound awareness and prosodic information, but she was unable to use them in understanding the speech of others. Technically, both Jenny and Bill are deaf in relation to their auditory capacities. But are the implications of their deafness also similar as they apply to their social, educational, and vocational futures?

About 1.7 million Americans are deaf under the criteria discussed above. About a quarter of these lost their hearing before the age of 19 (prevocationally deaf) and about half before the age of three (prelingually deaf). The implications of early deafness are serious in vocational planning because of speech and language deficiencies so often associated with this population. About 60% of employable deaf individuals hold skilled or semiskilled jobs. Another 20% do unskilled work, and less than 10% hold managerial or professional positions.

The intellectual capability of deaf individuals is no different from that of normally hearing subjects, as has been found in both quantitative and qualitative tests of performance. Deaf persons score less well, however, in cognitive tasks (learning rules, determining logical operations, sequential memory, etc.). The thought processes of some deaf people certainly may be affected by linguistic constraints, but it is also possible that they are limited by a reduced range of life experiences and the opportunity to learn therefrom.

The social patterns of deaf persons are relatively unique. Most of their social needs are met quite successfully within the deaf community in urban areas. They find acceptance, support, and the ability to communicate within this community—so much so that about 80% of them marry other deaf people. American Sign Language (ASL) is the common symbol system used for interhuman communication. Although increasing numbers of the hearing are learning ASL so that they might communicate more effectively with deaf individuals or provide interpretive services between deaf and hearing persons, there is still much to be done to break down the remaining barriers to human interaction.

It should be of no surprise that some deaf individuals develop personality problems and behavioral deficiencies as a result of reduced educational and social experiences that are taken for granted by hearing individuals. However, there is no evidence that the incidence of such problems is any higher than among hearing persons. The same can be said of more serious aspects of mental health, such as psychotic behavior.

Although those with usable hearing function (the hard-of-hearing) may experience problems vocationally, the primary effect of their loss is seen in behavioral changes that may occur in reaction to reduced communicative abilities. Changes in personality patterns are commonly associated with a slowly developing hearing impairment. In contrast to deaf individuals, who may find considerable social interaction in the deaf community, hearing-impaired persons sometimes develop a poor self-concept and feelings of inferiority if increasing communicative difficulties are constantly reinforced by negative experiences in social contacts with the hearing. They may respond by isolating themselves from such interactions as much as possible. This withdrawal behavior can lead to decreased human capacity in many ways, often resulting in serious misunderstandings within the constellation of family and friends. Even mild impairments in young children, if present for a sufficient period, can have serious implications for the development of speech and language and for general learning behavior. Resultant behavioral problems in the family are not uncommon, including social maladjustment in serious cases.

Not everyone with impaired hearing is confronted with educational, social, behavioral, and vocational problems such as those described above. Profoundly deaf persons typically find positive interpersonal and cultural relationships that are extremely rewarding. "Deaf Pride" and "Deaf Power" are concepts receiving wide recognition in the deaf community. Through the realization of their human and political potential, many deaf individuals are actively engaged in legislative efforts and educational activities designed to increase societal understanding and acceptance of their individual rights as a minority group. ASL instruction for hearing persons is becoming increasingly popular as artificial barriers to social interaction are being continually reduced. Communicative strategies are also increasing with the development of new electronic technology. TDDs (Telephone Devices for the Deaf), which allow messages to be typed, sent simultaneously by telephone, and received as a visual display in standard English, are becoming available throughout the professional and business world. And people with less severe impairments are finding that improved auditory and visual assistive devices are increasingly available in many physical settings. These developments are positive, indeed, and are in need of expansion throughout society. The primary determinant of effective human relationships is through a common language system that is adequately conveyed and perceived. *All* avenues of transmission—acoustic, visual, and tactile—should be readily available to ensure this goal.

Jenny and Bill are now 23-years-old. They were fortunate to have concerned, loving parents who obtained advice from others but still made their own decisions in the raising of their child.

Bill is attending Gallaudet University in Washington, D.C., where he is taking pre-engineering courses. He is also an active sprinter on the track team. Bill received his grade and high school education in a state school for the deaf, as had his parents. He has never worn a hearing aid, nor has he really had a desire to do so. He is perfectly satisfied with his ability to communicate effectively with his many colleagues and friends using ASL. He has a very positive self-image. He intends to find employment as an engineer and to marry another deaf person. His major frustration in life occurs in situations requiring use of written or spoken English, his second language. He continues to develop his written English skills and to speak and sign simultaneously, but is well aware that his speech articulation is not usually adequate in conversations with hearing listeners.

Jenny is about to graduate from the state university with a B.A. in education. She intends to enter graduate school and pursue a master's degree in education of the hearing impaired. Throughout her primary and secondary school years, Jenny received therapy focused on the maintenance of articulation skills that she can now monitor only by tactile sensations. Although some deterioration has occurred (intonation and some phonemic distortion and omission), her speech is quite intelligible. She has developed exceptional speechreading skills which, in combination with the tactile sensations provided by her hearing aids, allow her to communicate well with normal-hearing persons. Although Jenny's social life has not been as active as that of many of her hearing friends, she feels good about her accomplishments and the potential of her professional future. She has learned ASL and fingerspelling as tools she will need in teaching. Although she has not thought of herself as being "deaf," she has become increasingly interested in improving her new language skills while making new contacts with individuals in the local deaf community. She already feels fortunate that her communicative skills may eventually allow her to "bridge the gap" so that she might be a more effective communicator with all listeners, whether hearing or severely impaired.

Having considered the various descriptive categories and implications of hearing impairment, we will now address the strategies for its prevention and management. It is axiomatic that the most effective way to deal with hearing loss is to prevent it from occurring in the first place. Programs focused on this goal are common in populations identified as having a high potential for impaired hearing. In the next section we consider how efforts of this type are conducted and identify those individuals receiving primary attention in such programs.

HEARING CONSERVATION

Many of the disorders discussed in Chapter 8 can be prevented with appropriate sensitivity to impaired hearing as a social problem. Few would dispute the importance of public education in such efforts. Yet little attention is placed on the issue of hearing loss as a major issue. Why is this so? Perhaps it relates to the higher level in the "pecking order" assumed by other social ills, such as drugs, tobacco, poverty, and unemployment. Hearing loss is often looked upon as a slowly developing condition associated primarily with aging. Bleeding, pain, and discomfort are usually absent in adults. Consequently hearing loss has assumed a rather low priority as an issue deserving special effort (and funding) toward its prevention.

There are recent indications that this view may be changing, however. Evidence of public focus on specific noise problems in urban communities is appearing more frequently each year. Freeway and airport noise has become a major concern throughout the country. Legal action related to occupational noise exposure is more prevalent in the nation's courtrooms. And questions are being raised about individual noise exposure of young men and women in their recreational activities, such as the levels at which music is being produced for listening under stereo earphones and in enclosed spaces. The potential connection of permanent impairment with exposure to high sound intensities is more widely recognized now than ever before. Public awareness of this association is fundamental to hearing conservation, and the recognition that hearing loss can be prevented is also basic to any such plan.

Schools

Programs designed to identify hearing problems of young children have been actively pursued in the public schools for many years. All states mandate a hearing screening program of some type for all children in the early elementary grades. Such efforts have a dual purpose. The nation's education system is naturally concerned about potential learning disabilities that may be associated with impaired hearing in the school population, and children failing the tests in such screening programs are potential recipients of needed medical attention.

Few people in the United States progress through their early school years without experiencing a simple test of their hearing sensitivity. Screening audiometry usually consists of individual listening tests conducted under earphones. The child is presented with a series of three or four pure tones at a specific hearing level and is simply asked to respond each time the tone is heard. The frequencies usually include 1,000, 2,000, and 4,000 Hz; 500 and/or 3,000 Hz may also be used. The standard intensity may vary from 15 to 30 dB HL, depending on state regulations and the environmental test circumstances. Retests are normally administered at another time if a child is unresponsive to a signal. If the child fails the retest, threshold audiometry may then be conducted. The parents are usually notified, whether the results are abnormal or not. Medical referral may be recommended if it seems appropriate.

Some states in recent years have also introduced screening with immittance audiometry. Since this procedure is associated specifically with the physical condition of the ear rather than hearing sensitivity, its increasing popularity shows that school screening programs are paying closer attention to the medical implications of impaired hearing

The Urban Community

The intrusion of unwanted sound in our lives has been increasingly recognized over the last 20 years as an important social problem. Governmental action has resulted at a number of levels. As our society has become increasingly urbanized and populated, people in cities and suburban neighborhoods have been more concerned about the incursion of noise in their personal lives. Primary irritation has developed over aircraft and highway noise, especially among those living close to airports, freeways, and industrial areas. Barking dogs, the neighbor's power equipment (mowers, air conditioners, heat exchangers, audio amplifiers), intrusion of industrial and construction noise in the evening hours on the private property of others, transportation noise from many sources—all of these are examples of familiar noise sources in urban communities. Some experts believe that exposure to such noise over many years of urban living may contribute to decreased hearing in susceptible individuals. Such a condition has even been labeled: *sociocusis.*

Citizen complaints about community noise have been sufficient, in recent years, to warrant increased legislation at all levels of government. Ordinances regulating noise emissions and establishing maximum tolerable noise levels have been passed at city, county, and state levels throughout the country. The federal government has established regulations on airport and jet noise. Although these actions have led to improved environmental conditions in many instances, enforcement costs are high. As stated previously, expenditure of public taxes in this area has been a low priority. Consequently, sustained efforts at community noise prevention are often minimal. Enforcement tends to be reactive rather than proactive, initiated only after complaints are lodged about past exposures. Even so, the general public is becoming more cognizant of the problem. Periodic discussions in the media have sensitized potential noise polluters to public concern and have led to reductions of extraneous noise in some communities. Political entities, such as city and county health agencies, are often responsive to citizen complaints. But complaints must still be made.

Industry

Industrial noise has been recognized for decades as a major cause of permanent hearing impairment. The phrase "boiler-maker's deafness" was applied commonly in years past to describe a natural consequence of employment in the fabrication of large metal containers. Significant and permanent hearing loss was normally expected in many industrial settings, such as for sawyers in lumber mills and riveters in shipbuilding. There seemed to be no practical way to prevent it.

Early in 1950 it became clear that strategies were available to reduce the deleterious effects of industrial noise: hearing loss in such settings need not be an inevitability. The hearing sensitivity of employees can be monitored audiometrically so that appropriate actions can be initiated to protect those showing threshold changes from high exposure levels. Predominant noise sources can be identified with periodic noise surveys. In some cases, engineering controls can be applied to reduce the noise at the source. Hearing-protective devices, such as ear plugs and muffs, offer personal protection. Educational programs about hearing conservation can be initiated with both employer and employees.

Increased awareness that these protective strategies could be effective led to certain changes in worker's compensation regulations that began to appear in the 1950s. Each state developed monetary award formulas related to auditory threshold shifts thought to be a consequence of occupational exposure. As the worker nears retirement, successful demonstration of a permanent hearing loss *associated with past employment* can be compensated. But it soon became clear that *prevention* of such impairments not only was more cost-effective for employers and the government, but was a moral and legal responsibility of both. Consequently, some companies voluntarily initiated hearing conservation programs to educate their employees about the risks of noise exposure and established some or all of the conservation procedures mentioned above.

Federal regulations developed by the Occupational Safety and Health Administration (OSHA), Department of Labor, now specify that hearing conservation programs be established wherever dangerous noise levels occur during particular work periods. These approaches clearly mandate salutary environmental conditions for industrial employees. Unfortunately, as in the case of community noise, the effectiveness of these regulations is often limited by a lack of personnel and resources for proper inspection and enforcement.

MEDICAL MANAGEMENT

Many conditions causing hearing loss will occur, irrespective of whether viable hearing conservation programs are in place. Impaired function, in whatever system of the body it occurs, can be associated with a physical disorder having serious health consequences. As emphasized in Chapter 8, impaired hearing, tinnitus, and dizziness can be symptoms of disease processes needing immediate medical attention. Some conditions, such as hereditary abnormalities or degeneration associated with age, may not be amenable to medical or surgical intervention; but others, such as infectious disease and expanding tumors, may need urgent medical treatment as life-threatening conditions. A good management plan must always begin with a thorough consideration of the physical cause and the medical/surgical implications of the problem.

Once the cause of a hearing impairment is known, the physician formulates a treatment plan designed to alleviate the etiology and restore hearing function. Each of these worthy goals, of course, is qualified by how well medical or surgical intervention can correct the disorder. Generally, medical management incorporates three major approaches: chemical therapy using drugs, radiologic treatment, and surgical intervention. These strategies may be utilized singly or in various combinations according to the condition under treatment.

Infectious bacteria can usually be treated effectively with powerful antibiotics now available. Drugs may also be prescribed in certain vascular disorders to dilate tiny blood vessels or to prevent and/or dissolve clots. Diuretic medications, designed to decrease fluid content in body tissues, may reduce endolymphatic pressure in Meniere's disease. Antihistamines may be prescribed in allergic conditions, and various pain medications are helpful when needed. Clearly, many of the conditions related to disorders of the peripheral ear can be treated effectively through drug therapy.

Radiologic treatment may be selected for certain conditions in which abnormal cellular growth must be reduced or eliminated. These are usually benign or malignant tumors occurring in an area that cannot be reached or is not otherwise amenable to surgery. Often, however, such growths can be removed surgically, although impaired hearing may remain. A team composed of an otologist and a neurosurgeon sometimes performs this delicate work.

Surgery is also the treatment of choice in certain conditions of the middle ear in which the normal transformer function has been compromised. Plastic repair of residual damage to the tympanic membrane and/or ossicles is called *tympanoplasty*. After a chronic infection has been medically treated, surgical reconstruction may improve mechanical function in the middle ear, leading to better energy flow into the cochlea and improved hearing. Surgery may also provide a new ear canal in cases of congenital maldevelopment.

The common childhood condition of middle-ear fluid accumulation is often treated by making a small incision in the tympanic membrane (a *myringotomy*) and inserting a tiny plastic tube into the opening (Fig. 9.1). This device may remain in place for six months or longer. Its presence maintains pressure equalization between the outer and middle ears until normal function of the auditory tube is restored. If fluid exists at the time of surgery, it can be removed with suction during the procedure.

Timmy, aged four, had experienced periodic infections in each ear in the last two years. Frequent trips to the doctor with a very unhappy boy were not an uncommon experience for his parents. Antibiotic treatment was often sufficient to alleviate the bacterial infection, but it was clear to the physician that Timmy's tonsils and adenoids were enlarged

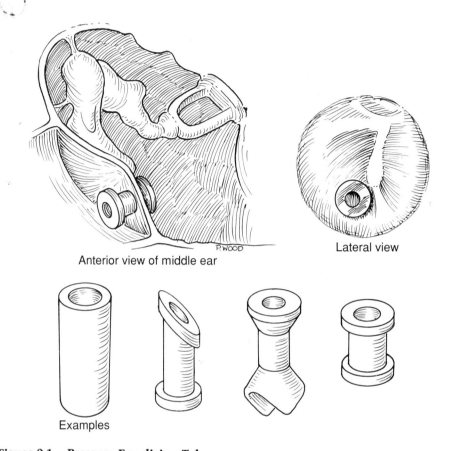

Anterior view of middle ear

Lateral view

Examples

Figure 9.1. Pressure-Equalizing Tubes
The tube is inserted in a myringotomy opening; its resulting position in the tympanic membrane is shown. Various types of tubes are illustrated.

and likely contributed to poor auditory-tube function. Following removal of the tonsils and adenoids under general anesthesia, a myringotomy was performed in each ear with extraction of residual middle-ear fluid. A small pressure-equalization tube was then inserted in the eardrum opening to ensure that negative middle-ear pressure would not occur during the period that normal auditory-tube function was developing. Both of the tubes were removed in five months, and the small hole in the tympanic membrane closed spontaneously in a few days. Timmy's hearing was restored to normal, and earaches were no longer a part of his life.

One of the most successful surgical approaches to hearing restoration is a technique called *stapedectomy.* This procedure is employed in the treatment of otosclerosis. While viewing the ear through a microscope, the surgeon cuts the canal skin around a portion of the tympanic membrane so that the membrane can be retracted and the middle-ear cavity viewed directly. After the presence of the oto-sclerotic growth is confirmed, the stapes and accompanying footplate are completely removed. Ossicular chain continuity is restored with a tiny prosthesis; the materials used depend on the surgeon's choice. One combination is a small plastic tube inserted between the incus and a tiny piece of vein (from elsewhere in the patient's body) that is placed across the oval window opening. Another is a wire attached to the incus and connected to a small piece of fat or inert plastic covering the window. A third system is a tiny piston made of steel or teflon that is attached to the incus and moves in and out of a hole created in the oval window. All of these approaches have the same general result: the integrity of the ossicular chain is restored, and sounds may now enter the cochlea in an effective manner. The procedure is usually done under a local anesthetic. The patient often notices an immediate hearing improvement on the operating table. In many cases, hearing sensitivity is shortly restored to the normal range.

Another surgical approach of recent years is that associated with the *cochlear implant* (Fig. 9.2). This procedure is being used in selected individuals having severe to profound hearing impairment and who cannot utilize hearing aids effectively. A wire with one or more tiny electrodes is inserted into the cochlea through the round window and is then attached to a magnetic receiver embedded in the mastoid bone behind the ear. Sounds are processed by an externally worn device driving a magnetic transmitter placed on the skin over the implanted receiver. The processed sound is magnetically induced into the implant. The intention is that this energy will stimulate any functional nerve endings remaining in the peripheral system. Although recipients of these devices do not experience normal hearing for speech, increased sound awareness of the acoustic environment usually does occur. An intensive educational and auditory training program is conducted following the implantation to relate new auditory experiences with associated auditory stimuli and to enhance the effectiveness of visual cues.

AUDIOLOGIC MANAGEMENT

Audiologic approaches to improved hearing are focused on strategies for maximizing speech recognition. Attention is placed on increased receptivity of speech cues through amplification and visual observation. Specialized educational techniques are used to improve the simultaneous perception of amplified sound in association with cues provided by the speaker's bodily and facial movements and by the situational context of the conversation. Those profiting from such approaches must, of course, have residual hearing function and good visual acuity. These programs are referred to as aural rehabilitation (for those who have lost auditory function that once was present) or aural habilitation (for those impaired at birth or before oral language skills were developed).

Hearing Aids

Increasing sound intensity, by whatever means, would appear to be the most satisfactory means of overcoming hearing impairment—simply make sound louder

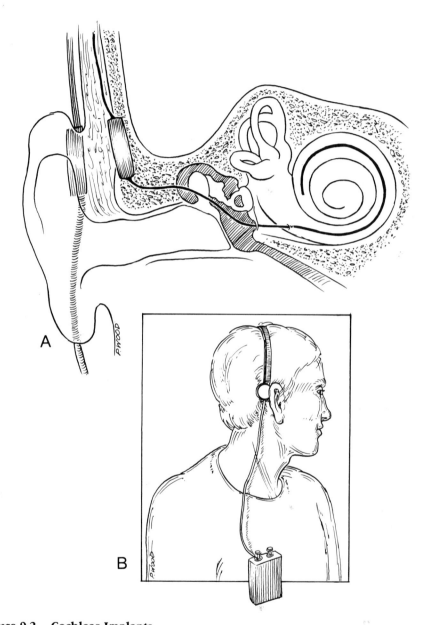

Figure 9.2.   Cochlear Implants
A, a wire is surgically threaded into the cochlea and is connected to an induction coil situated just below the skin. **B,** a second coil is worn over the first, inducing sounds processed by the stimulator worn on the body.

and the "loss" wil be eliminated. For some, such an approach is completely satisfactory in restoring both sensitivity and intelligibility. For others it may help, but speech intelligibility may still be poor without supplementation through other approaches.

Aids to hearing occur everywhere and are used commonly by normal listeners in difficult situations. Turning up the volume on the television, stereo, or radio can be an effective way for the hearing-impaired person to compensate for a loss and for the normally hearing individual to overcome extraneous noise in the environment. Both may profit by asking others to talk louder. Moving into a quiet environment can aid hearing by eliminating unnecessary acoustic distraction. Cupping the hand behind the pinna often helps, especially in improving reception for high-frequency sounds. Even ear trumpets that concentrate sound energy at the ear canal were of help in the past.

Modern electronic hearing aids are miniature amplifiers built into a small, wearable package that is aestetically acceptable to the potential wearer. The amplification process is basically similar in all hearing aids (Fig. 9.3). A tiny microphone and associated circuitry, driven by a battery of less than 2 volts, transpose acoustic signals into electronic energy. Transistors and other components amplify the power of the electrical stimulus; this is then converted back to sound by another microphone, the receiver, which operates like a miniature loudspeaker. The receiver is directly coupled to the ear. A volume or gain control is usually provided to regulate intensity. Some instruments also provide controls to amplify certain frequencies more than others (i.e., tone control) and to regulate the maximum decibel output (gain) of the aid. Certain aids are equipped with special coils so that they can be inductively coupled to a telephone receiver, often providing a signal of higher fidelity than through the acoustic pathway. Environmental noise in the room is not amplified using this device, and intelligibility can be considerably improved.

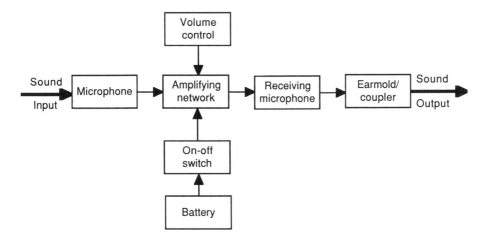

Figure 9.3. Schematic of Hearing Aid Components
Instruments not worn "in the ear" are "coupled" to the canal with an earmold. Most instruments sold today are actually built into the coupler/earmold itself.

Electronic technology now allows this circuitry to be encased in a variety of packages, some of which are quite small (Fig. 9.4). Most of the instruments sold today are worn entirely in the ear canal opening (in-the-ear, or ITE) or in the canal itself (ITC). Some are even built into the temple pieces of eyeglasses. Others may be worn immediately behind the pinna (behind-the-ear, or BTE aids). Some persons with severe impairments still use instruments carried in a shirt pocket, in a halter, or in some other manner on the body. Amplified sound is then carried through a cord to an external receiver worn at the ear. Less than 1% of hearing aids sold in the United States in 1988 were body aids, however; over 79% of aids sold were ITE or ITC instruments.

An impression of part of the ear canal and pinna configuration must be made for the ear being "fitted." From this impression, a plastic earmold is constructed. The function of the mold will depend on the type of aid to be worn. If it is a body aid, the earmold will hold the external receiver in place; if a BTE aid, a plastic tube from the aid's internal receiver is inserted into the earmold; and if an ITE aid, the electronic components are inserted into the earmold shell, which then fits entirely within the ear opening and canal.

Since hearing aids are so small, their amplifying capacity is necessarily limited to the frequency range of speech sounds that have been impaired. The majority of

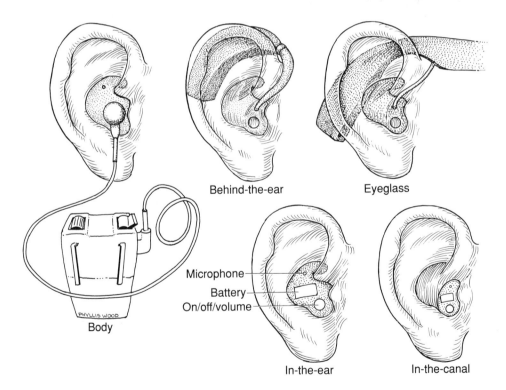

Behind-the-ear   Eyeglass

Microphone
Battery
On/off/volume

Body

In-the-ear   In-the-canal

Figure 9.4. Examples of Hearing Aid Styles

persons wearing aids are those who develop a sensorineural loss in the higher frequencies later in life. Consequently, most instruments are designed to provide the greatest gain for frequencies between 1,000 and 3,500 Hz.

The first question to be asked when considering hearing aids in a person's management plan is whether there is good reason to expect them to be helpful. In some ways, "the best hearing aid is the one that is worn." Using such instruments is a voluntary act; few individuals do so unless they experience improved audition. How, then, does one know that a hearing aid (or two, for that matter) will be worth the cost? And which make and model among the hundreds on the market will be "the best" for a particular person?

Predicting successful use of hearing aids is an inexact endeavor, often depending on personal and emotional factors important to the prospective wearer. The societal bias against hearing aids so common in the past is still an important consideration for some, but is less of an obstacle in recent years. Acceptance of hearing aids has been enhanced by their reduced size and by the recent popularization of hearing-aid wear associated with former-President Reagan's use of canal aids.

Generally, the person profiting most by hearing aids is the conductively impaired. As stated in Chapter 8, the major need here is in only one dimension: improved sound intensity. Once speech is amplified by the aid, the normal sensorineural system can process it effectively in most cases. But very few individuals with conductive impairments need to wear hearing aids since medical and/or surgical treatment usually solves their problem.

One exception to the last statement is represented by Tammy. She was born with small stubs of cartilage on each side of her head where the pinnae normally belong. In addition, she had no ear canals. Because of arrested fetal development, her external ear was completely obstructed by bone. Although plastic surgery might be considered for her at a later age when her skull reached an appropriate size, it was clear that she desperately needed some alternative means to bring sound into her normally functional sensorineural system.

After a number of tests confirmed that she could respond to sound by bone conduction, two body-style instruments were placed in halters strapped to her chest. Each instrument activated a bone-conduction oscillator held by a specially designed headband to each side of her head. For the first time she began to associate the sounds of her mother's voice with the smiling face she had observed during her first six months. Some sounds, at first, were disruptive since they had no meaning. But soon Tammy began the language-learning process natural to all hearing children—exploring the sounds of her own vocal babbling and associating the myriad auditory stimuli of her environment with the visual and tactile world around her.

But what of those with sensorineural impairments—the ability to process speech when it is sufficiently loud to overcome their sensitivity loss, but with considerable distortion of the signal by the time it reaches the brain? Remember that many of these listeners are confronted with lowered tolerance to loud sound, sometimes compounding their receptive problem.

The auditory difficulties associated with sensorineural impairment have, in the past, led to some negative opinions about the use of hearing aids. Typical assumptions were that one must have a moderate to severe loss to be a possible candidate and that speech intelligibility would still be insufficient to warrant the cost of the instrument. The experiences of most hearing-aid users today, however, support a much more positive view. The wide range of electroacoustic variables available in modern hearing instruments ensures a higher potential for meeting the unique needs of individuals with losses of all degrees. When coupled with strategies for improved listening and visual skills that can be learned by the hearing impaired, the majority of those with residual hearing capacity can be significantly assisted with wearable amplification.

The audiologist uses a number of tests to predict the need for amplification and whether speech recognition will improve sufficiently to warrant its use. These tests are done at threshold and suprathreshold levels, with and without hearing aids, to determine the optimum gain characteristics, frequency response, and maximum allowable output required in each case. The closest match is then made between these requirements and the electroacoustic properties of specific instruments available to the dispenser in an acceptable package. Final acceptance of any recommended instrument(s) often awaits a short trial period by the listener, who must (and should) make the ultimate decision.

Once it is determined that amplification is a desirable alternative, multiple questions must be answered. Which of the various types (BTE, ITE, ITC, body, eyeglass) will be acceptable to the listener and still offer the necessary electroacoustic characteristics? In which ear should it be worn, or should two aids be used? Should special features be included, such as a telephone coil? If the listener is a small child, will a special halter or headband be necessary to maintain the aid comfortably and safely on the body or head?

> At 68 years of age, Bob was still an active and reasonably successful salesman. But he was aware that his hearing had been changing for the worse in the previous three or four years. His wife and family members were asking whether his ears were alright, since he asked for repetitions in family conversations. He also liked the television volume turned higher than did other family members, and he often did not respond to his wife's call from another room. He even missed telephone rings from time to time. But of even greater concern was the fact that his customers were drawing his attention to errors he was making in orders received over the telephone.
>
> Bob's physician sent him to an otologist, who confirmed that his loss was associated with aging and that no medical or surgical intervention was warranted. An audiologist then found that Bob had a mild to moderate high-frequency sensorineural loss in both ears and that his speech discrimination was reasonably good with sufficient amplification. The emphasis provided by instruments worn in each ear canal provided substantial compensation for his high-frequency loss. His speech intelligibility was considerably enhanced when wearing the aids, including telephone use. Bob was pleased to recognize again such sounds as bird calls and rustling leaves that had been missing from his listening repertoire for some time.

Another benefit of hearing-aid wear is sometimes noted by persons with tinnitus. When the aid is on, the tinnitus may be significantly diminished, or completely eliminated in some cases; the intensity of amplified sound is sufficient to "mask out" the wearer's tinnitus. Some tinnitus sufferers have also found relief by using instruments with noise makers built into a hearing-aid package (usually worn behind the ear). These devices produce a constant noise in the ear, sounding something like "shhhhhhhh." Sounds can still enter the ear canal normally so that lower frequencies can be heard. One might think that such a noise would be annoying to the wearer, but those who find the device useful claim that their tinnitus may be effectively reduced or eliminated—a result that is sufficiently desirable to make the masker an acceptable part of their listening experience.

Hearing aids are dispensed by many audiologists in community, medical, educational, and private practice settings. They may also be purchased from dispensers who are not clinical audiologists, but who have met licensure requirements established by most states (as have dispensing audiologists). The cost of individual aids is variable, but typically ranges between $400 and $800.

Assistive Listening Devices

A wide variety of electronic amplifiers have become available in recent years that are used by hard-of-hearing individuals in specific listening situations. Some may substitute for personal hearing aids, and others may actually be coupled to the listener's own aid.

One of the more obvious examples is a telephone amplifier that can be purchased for home or office use. It can be set at desirable levels by a separate gain control in the handset. Such devices may provide up to 30% more power for the listener. Portable amplifiers are also available that can be carried from place to place. These instruments are attached to a regular telephone handset for increased amplification. They are not compatible with all telephone models, however. Amplifier headsets are also being installed at public telephones in hotels, transportation facilities, and even street kiosks. They are usually identified by an appropriate symbol indicating that the telephone has amplifying capability for the hearing impaired.

Audio signals are also enhanced in various ways for group listening in large rooms. The *audio loop system* consists of a microphone and amplifier attached to a length of wire that is "looped" around the seating area. The current passing through the wire establishes a magnetic field that can be picked up by some hearing aids or special receivers worn by the listener sitting in the loop. Another device employs a regular *AM system* similar to a radio that transmits only the desired sound to individually worn sets. And a third, not surprisingly, compromises an *FM system* that also delivers sound to an individual receiver or to some hearing aids with a special attachment. An advantage of the latter two is that the listener is not physically restricted to a defined area, as is necessary with the loop system. The audio systems are often employed in school programs for the hearing impaired.

The development of *infrared technology* has significantly increased the variety of wireless devices available for use in large auditoria. Sound from the public address system is transmitted by infrared light emitters in the form of harmless light rays. These signals are received by personally worn devices that convert the rays into amplified sound and convey it to the ears of the listener. These instruments, as well as hard-wired systems, can be worn in the home for listening to television and conversation.

New electronic technology provides enormous communicative enhancement to deaf people and to those who have hearing but desire a more effective means of personal contact with deaf persons. The *TDD*, mentioned earlier, is an instrument that looks something like a typewriter keyboard. A cradle for the handset of a telephone is provided so that once the connection is made between two individuals, telecommunication can be established by the transmission and reception of specific sounds associated with letters and numbers. Each word typed on the keyboard is instantaneously displayed by the device; some even include a printer for a permanent copy of the conversation. The instruments use a dedicated telephone line. If the person being contacted, such as a physician, does not have a TDD, the caller can communicate through a message-relay operator in many communities. The operator will dial the number desired and then convert print to voice and vice versa.

Various alternating systems for the hearing impaired have also been developed in recent years. Amplified audio alarms, bright and blinking lights, and even tactile stimulators are now available to signal the sound of doorbells, telephone rings, baby cries, and paging devices, and the onset of security, wake-up, and smoke alarms. Some electronic pagers utilize both sound and vibration and will provide printed data indicating who should be called.

All of these developments have significantly increased the personal contact of severely hearing impaired persons with their surrounding world. The devices may be purchased from many telephone retail stores and from specialty shops dealing specifically with assistive listening devices and their installation. Assistive input is not limited to electronic technology, however. Dogs have been recruited; they are of enormous help in alerting their owners to environmental sound. The animals are being trained to "announce" such sounds as door and telephone bells, knocking, the whistle of a tea kettle, audible fire alarms, etc. These stimuli and many others become the repertoire of sound-alerting used by the "hearing aid" dog.

Auditory Training

Children who wear hearing aids for the first time are often puzzled by the new sounds in their lives. Since these sounds have little meaning, they may initially represent little more than unwanted noise. The children must learn to recognize the value of these new sounds, or the hearing aid could be rejected. Formal educational activities designed to assist them in this task are often initiated shortly after the aid is obtained. Attention is focused on the meaning of the new sounds in the child's life—

the relationship of amplified sound to animals, people, and items of interest in the environment. As the child's awareness to these stimuli is increased, the ability to discriminate their unique spectral characteristics is improved. This process develops into recognition of the rhythmic characteristics of speech—the stress patterns and intonation used by talkers in the child's surroundings. And as the child learns to imitate these new sounds and to observe the reactions of others to this expressive behavior, language develops and new speech skills are learned.

Such educational programs may be conducted in structured sessions by audiologists and speech-language pathologists in preschool or community service settings. Since parents often are effective educators, they should become active participants in this new learning activity. Strategies can be taught to the parents that include listening and sound-identifying games. In some localities, audiologists spend short periods in the home with the parents and preschoolers, demonstrating educational techniques that help the child distinguish among environmental and speech sounds under aided conditions.

Generally, these activities center around sound recognition games, starting with rather gross stimuli (such as recordings of automobiles, a dog barking, water pouring, bells ringing, etc.) and leading to the identification of more subtle sound differences, including individual phonemes, spoken words, and sentences. After it is clear that the child is able to use the hearing aid(s) effectively in detecting the speech of others, sentence identification may be stressed. After various sentences are created that describe a known object or event, the child learns to utilize acoustic cues in correctly choosing the appropriate sentence without the benefit of visual input. The same may be done using words—helping the child to distinguish between those having different stress patterns (fish, baseball, turtle) and gradually working into discriminating among words of similar temporal patterns (ice cream, hot dog, toothbrush). The ultimate objective of such learning, of course, is maximizing the capability of the child to understand audible speech.

The involvement of the parents in this activity is often helpful as a coping strategy, since many parents go through a natural "grieving" period once they learn of their child's impairment. Participation in habilitative learning activities such as this can lead them into more positive attitudes toward themselves and the capabilities of their child.

Activities focused on amplified sound recognition can also be of assistance for some adults in the early stages of hearing-aid wear. Lessons on the acoustic recognition of speech sounds, through hearing aids and telephone amplifiers, can be of considerable help in relearning speech intelligibility skills that once were automatically available. Simple listening strategies can be discussed with the new hearing-aid wearer at the time the aid is dispensed. They include ways in which more complex listening situations can be approached slowly after the listener is acquainted with amplified sounds under controlled circumstances, such as in the home. Orientation periods can also provide the audiologist with an opportunity to evaluate the individual's need for specialized attention to visual cues in speech communication.

Speechreading

Many hearing-impaired persons develop exceptional skill in supplementing imperfect auditory information with visual cues obtained from the facial expressions and general bodily movements of the speaker. At times, this skill is developed almost on a subconscious level by persons who lose their hearing slowly. Attention is focused not just on the lips of the speaker, but on the total visual experience associated with the speech process. For this reason, the word "speechreading" is preferred over "lipreading" as a name for this receptive skill. Visual observations can provide valuable information regarding the speaker's emotional state, the context and meaning of the message, and specific speech sounds that might not have been heard accurately.

Many of the sounds of speech are readily observed by the average listener. They are referred to as *visemes*, meaning visual phonemes. These include the sounds /p/, /b/, and /m/; /f/, /v/, /s/, and /t/; and /w/. Even /k/ and /g/ are included, in certain word positions. One must remember that these visemes do not occur in isolation, but as parts of continuous speech. Even the identification of individual words by visual means is inexact because so many words are *homophenous*. These are words having the same general appearance on the lips, such as "mud" and "mutt", "but" and "been"; "pint" and "bite"; etc. But highly visible phonemes represent, at best, only about 40% of the speech sounds normally used in speech communication. The others, such as most of the vowels and many of the remaining consonants, are not easily observed. Fortunately, however, the vowel sounds are easier to hear since they contain relatively more sound energy in the lower frequencies.

Audiologists and speech-language pathologists provide lessons designed to improve speechreading skills for those sufficiently motivated to learn such observational techniques. These lessons are often combined with exercises in auditory training during the early stages of wearing a new hearing aid. Educational strategies with hearing-impaired children usually incorporate speechreading and auditory training activities with lessons in language learning.

Training in speechreading ordinarily involves formalized lessons designed to increase awareness of useful nonverbal cues in the environment. These observations are related to the information being communicated orally. The listener must develop high sensitivity for other nonauditory cues. These include attention to the linguistic and situational information contained in all oral communication. The structure of language provides rules that narrow the options available when certain words, sounds, or phrases are not heard, and the situation and context of the message also reduce the number of possibilities for word/sound closure. In addition to improved visual perception, speechreading instruction focuses on the development of visual concentration and a longer attention span.

For some, the task of mastering these skills is achieved rather quickly; for others, it requires extensive practice and personal discipline. Success is often tied directly to the motivation of the client and the ability of the clinician to maintain a positive attitude toward the activity and the outcome. For these reasons, formalized lessons in speechreading and auditory training often involve groups of hearing-impaired persons who can share their experiences, are mutually supportive, and provide the humor and personal interchange that make social encounters more satisfying.

EDUCATIONAL CONSIDERATIONS

Perhaps the greatest challenge in responding to the special needs of the hearing impaired is associated with the development of language and of effective methods for communicating linguistic concepts to others. Such a goal is clearly attainable in most individuals who develop even severely impaired hearing, *if* the onset follows a period of normal hearing and speech/language learning early in life. But for those who are prelingually impaired (during the first three years or at birth), the implications of even a moderate loss can be serious, and they become almost overwhelming when the degree of impairment is profound. The differences between the hearing and the prelingually deaf child in this context have been described by Moores (1987, p. 3):[1]

"Children with normal hearing can be considered linguistically proficient in every sense of the word. They have a knowledge of the basic rules of their language. They can produce a potentially infinite number of novel yet appropriate utterances. Because of their unconscious mastery over the grammatical structure of their language, they can combine and recombine its elements indefinitely. They can produce and understand sentences to which they have never been exposed. They enter the formal educational situation in elementary school around age six with a fully developed instrument for learning: language and communication ability—an ability that they have acquired with no conscious effort on the part of their parents or themselves.

"By contrast, profoundly deaf children usually present an entirely different picture. Unless they have deaf parents, they probably have not acquired a language naturally and automatically. Without intensive compensatory training they may be totally nonverbal as well as nonvocal; they even may be unaware that such things as words exist. For such children language is not a facilitating device for the acquisition of knowledge. Rather it is a barrier standing between them and the full realization of their academic, intellectual, and social potentials. Typical deaf children, although of normal intelligence, find their range of experience constrained by communication limitations. They suffer, relative to other children, from a lack of opportunity to interact fully with and manipulate their environment in meaningful ways. Although deafness itself may have no effect on intellectual potential, the deafness will lead to impoverished communication skills that themselves may limit develoment severely, unless the children are provided compensatory tools."

Educational Settings

Once an impairment is confirmed and general information about its degree and nature is known, early planning of the child's special needs is imperative. There can be no excuse for delay; the child must be provided with every opportunity for language

---

[1]From Moores, Donald I. (1987). *Educating the Deaf,* 3rd ed. Boston: Houghton Mifflin. © 1987, Houghton Mifflin Company. Used with permission.

learning and speech development. Hearing-aid amplification should be given serious consideration. The parents of preschool-aged children must learn special strategies for enhanced oral communication that can be used in the home. In many localities, specialized programs are available that provide instructional materials for parents and periodic home visits by audiologists and special educators for consultations. Eventually, however, the child will be ready for placement in a formal program for hearing-impaired children.

The selection of an appropriate educational setting is not a simple decision. Although practical considerations such as cost, geographic location, and transportation may play important roles, the best decisions are based on two primary knowledge bases: a thorough understanding of the child's unique needs and awareness of the educational service facilities and personnel available to meet these needs. Parents usually lack sufficient information to make these judgments independently. In urban communities, consultation is normally provided by many agencies serving the needs of communicatively impaired children and adults. These include community and university speech and hearing centers, hospital clinics, governmental health agencies, and special education services in the schools.

If the child's aided hearing is reasonably good and the impairment occurred postlingually, the necessary specialized educational intervention may be minimal. Supplementary instruction in speech articulation, auditory training, and speechreading, provided periodically by speech-language pathologists in a regular school setting, may be quite adequate for such a child.

But much more specialized intervention is necessary for the more than 50,000 school-aged children in the United States who are deaf or whose aided hearing is inappropriate to their oral language capability. Until about 15 years ago, formal educational programs for these children were primarily limited to privately operated day-school or residential programs requiring, in many cases, significant financial support from the parents. An alternative choice has been residential placement in schools for deaf children that were established by state legislatures many years ago and are publicly funded. Parents who would have preferred having their children living at home during their school years often had little choice but to utilize residential institutions since day-school placement either was not available locally or was financially prohibitive.

In 1975, Congress passed Public Law 94-142, otherwise known as the "Education for All" act. This legislation mandates that all handicapped children shall be provided with a free, appropriate public education whether in the regular public school system or by contract to alternative resources when not available in the schools. Additionally, an Individualized Education Plan must be established annually for each designated child. The plan is prepared by appropriate professionals in the educational environment and is approved by the parents.

This act has been responsible for an enormous expansion of educational services for children having all degrees of hearing impairment and ranging from preschool age to 19 years. New programs, most involving day-school placements, have been established in almost all urban school districts. Specialized personnel in deaf education, working with professionals in school psychology, audiology, speech-language pathology, and vocational/educational counseling, are involved in these efforts. Almost 10,000 qualified teachers of deaf children have been educated in over 70 colleges and universities in the United States to provide for the specialized instructional needs of these children.

What potential has been available to the young deaf adult in achieving the intellectual and vocational benefits of a higher education? Until recent years, such opportunities were extremely limited. Gallaudet University in Washington, DC, is still the only liberal arts college for the deaf in the world. This institution, created by Congress in 1864, offers a regular four-year undergraduate degree in many disciplines and graduate programs in some areas. Students are selected on a competitive basis from applicants throughout the country. Approximately 1,000 are enrolled each year. The university also operates model educational programs at the primary and secondary levels for hearing-impaired children and conducts clinical and research programs in the communication sciences and disorders. Another institution, also established and maintained by Congress, was opened in 1968. The National Technical Institute for the Deaf is affiliated with the Rochester, New York, Institute of Technology. Its educational focus is oriented more toward advanced technical and vocational education. It also maintains an active research program that has provided new insights into communication modes used by deaf persons and the application of new technology to deaf education. Other vocational programs for young deaf adults have been supported by the federal government throughout the country.

Recent sensitivity to the needs of handicapped adults has significantly enhanced educational opportunities for deaf adults in public and private universities. Few deaf individuals have been able to utilize such institutions in the past because of the obvious communicative barriers. Appropriate support services, funded from public and private sources, are now available for deaf students in many of these public institutions. Such services may include manual interpreting, note taking, tutoring, social and vocational counseling, and supplementary instruction in communication skills. The need for more hearing personnel to provide such services has led to new professional training programs for interpreters throughout the country. Professional interpreters are also providing the communicative link between deaf and hearing persons in medical environments, in the courts and legal profession, and in many businesses.

Modes of Communication

In what manner should a teacher, whether hearing or impaired, communicate with a deaf child? And how should the child respond, especially if deafened prelinguistically?

The answers to these important questions have been debated among parents, special educators, and deaf individuals for many years. Four communicative modes receive primary attention today, each having numerous adherents and detractors. The *oral* approach is based on the position that natural language learning and speech expression is so much a part of "normal" functioning in society that it should be the only acceptable communicative avenue. The focus is on maximal utilization of whatever residual hearing remains to the child and on the supplementary visual cues associated with the speech act. Oral speech is the only mode of expression; the receptive avenue combines enhanced speechreading skills with hearing-aid amplification. The use of manual sign systems as a communicative tool is rejected; it is considered a distractor in the learning of oral speech and language.

A variation of the oral method is that proposed by the *auditory* school. This unisensory approach also supports oral speech expression, but emphasizes the hearing channel over visual recognition skills as the primary receptive mode. Speechreading, writing, and reading take a secondary role to the development of listening skills. For obvious reasons, this approach is used more with children having moderate losses than with profoundly deaf children.

A third approach (the *Rochester* method) combines speech expression and receptive skills through the auditory and speechreading channels with fingerspelling. Emphasis is placed on reading, writing, and speaking; both teacher and student employ oral speech simultaneously with spelling of individual words using the manual alphabet (Fig. 9.5).

The *simultaneous* method is, perhaps, the most eclectic of the four since it combines the oral method with fingerspelling and signed English. Although oral speech is used as much as possible in both expressive and receptive contexts, attention is focused on all avenues that might effectively be utilized in language learning and the expression of ideas. The term *total communication* is often used as an alternative designation for this method. This approach seems to be receiving increased support, especially in the education of young children. Motivation for this method has been based on such factors as a growing acceptance of the language of signs in society, general dissatisfaction with other methods, and the apparent support of deaf adults for this approach.

Consideration of Speech Deficits

An appropriate treatment plan for hard-of-hearing persons must be sensitive to oral expressive skills as well as audition. The needs of each person will, in the main, be dependent on the degree and the onset time of the impairment. Once adequate speech skills are developed using an intact feedback loop provided by functional audition, vision, and touch, deterioration in vocal and articulatory mannerisms can easily occur with an acquired hearing impairment. This is true for a child of seven years as well as an adult of 65. Although speech behaviors will vary under these conditions, expressive speech may begin to sound like that being heard by the hearing-impaired person. Sounds of low energy and high frequency, such as the sibilants and fricatives, may be distorted or even missing. If the hearing loss is sufficiently severe, voice quality and intonation may become inappropriate—vocal intensity may decrease and inflectional patterns may be changed.

Measures designed to sensitize a person to these possibilities and to teach

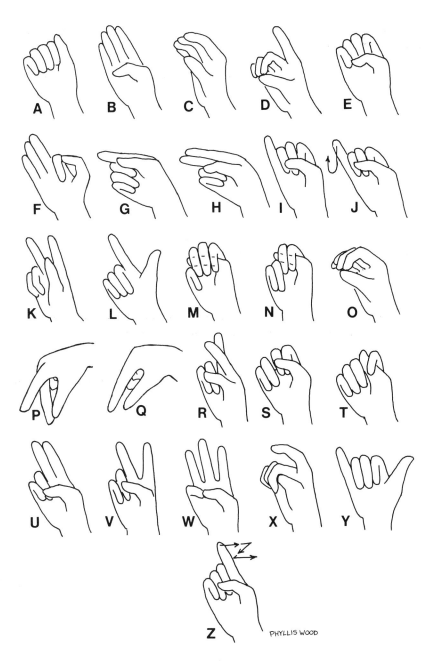

Figure 9.5. The American Manual Alphabet.
Seen from the visual perspective of the observer. All positions are static except those for *J* and *Z*.

strategies that might reduce their occurrence are often referred to as *speech conservation techniques.* Emphasis is placed on increased awareness of kinesthetic cues as the articulators and larynx are properly positioned. Tactile and visual feedback channels must supplement whatever audition remains. For these reasons, work on expressive speech skills is usually combined with speechreading and auditory training activities in many rehabilitative programs. Such services are often provided by speech-language pathologists as well as audiologists.

LOCAL AND NATIONAL RESOURCES

Those who are specially educated as service providers for hard-of-hearing and deaf persons have been identified throughout this chapter and in Chapter 8. Otologists, audiologists, hearing-aid dispensers, speech-language pathologists, teachers of the hearing impaired, vocational and psychological counselors—all are ready to assist as needed. But how does one know which discipline is needed, and where are such specialists found?

Since impaired hearing involves physical dysfunction, the first approach should be a medical one. Depending on the nature of the problem, such an avenue might be the only choice necessary. The family physician will be a helpful resource in choosing an otologic specialist, should one be needed. Such specialists are also listed in the yellow pages under "physicians/otology." They may also be located by calling the local medical society.

But what if medical or surgical therapy is unsuccessful in restoring function or if it is not appropriate treatment? Otologists should be aware of nonmedical services available locally and make appropriate referrals. In the absence of such advice, where might further information be obtained and services provided?

Intelligent choices can best be made only after adequate knowledge is provided to the impaired person or the parent/guardian. The information must clarify the nature of the problem, its potential impact on the individual, and where appropriate resources can be found for help. One might look, again, at the yellow pages. For those living in a large urban community, individuals and agencies listing services related to impaired hearing may be found under such designations as "audiologists" and "hearing aids." If one lives in a rural community, such listings may not be available. Travel to a larger population center may be mandatory.

If a young child is thought to be impaired, or a loss develops adventitiously in a child or adult and cannot be medically treated, audiologic evaluation and counseling are usually the first step in developing an effective management plan. The audiologist's skill in evaluating auditory function will provide an understanding of how much hearing is available to the individual and the potential of audiologic habilitative/rehabilitative strategies in each case. This information is conveyed in detail, and suggestions are then made as to the local resources that can be of assistance. These might include hearing-aid procurement; consultation regarding speechreading, auditory training, and speech conservation; psychologic and educational counseling; and advice on special educational facilities from which parents must make a choice.

Audiologic services may be found in a variety of settings. Audiologists may be private practitioners, and sometimes they are associated with otologic practices. They may also be located in large hospitals, in community speech and hearing centers, and in clinics operated by colleges and universities. Governmental agencies, such as the Veterans Administration, utilize extensive audiologic services. School programs specializing in the educational needs of hearing-impaired and deaf children often have the services of an audiologist.

In urban communities, many specialized services are becoming increasingly available for deaf adults and for the parents of deaf children. These facilities, usually in community colleges or service centers, provide social, educational, psychologic, and vocational counseling. Governmental agencies for crippled children, vocational rehabilitation, and services for the aged can also be of significant help. Often an excellent source of information about deafness and the services provided by professionals and service agencies in local communities can be found by simply contacting those national organizations dedicated to providing further information on impaired hearing and disorders of communication (see Appendix).

SUMMARY

Hearing impairment, in its many forms, can have widely varying impacts on the lives of those so impaired and on those with whom they come in contact. For some, the pathway to satisfactory hearing restoration is relatively short. Medical treatment, surgical intervention, hearing-aid amplification, aural/visual training—these approaches can lead to the capability of effective oral communication in many cases. But for others, oral speech and the auditory system may never be used to the satisfaction of either speaker or listener. Alternative strategies may be necessary, including different systems of symbolizing ideas and concepts.

Whatever the individual's needs might be, they must be identified as soon as possible. Following medical and audiologic evaluation, a plan of action must be established. The impaired individual and significant others must become maximally informed so that decisions regarding management alternatives are not delayed. For children, such considerations are vital in language learning and educational/social development. In the older person, they can lead to positive coping strategies and communicative skills that provide improved self-esteem and social interaction.

As more opportunities arise for interaction between the hearing and those with hearing loss, we should see increased understanding about deafness and its consequences. And with knowledge will come improved ways to exchange ideas. There is still much to be done. Many alternatives are not achieved because of financial limitations. Hearing aids are not provided under Medicare. Decisions on the education of some children are being made on the basis of financial or geographic considerations rather than the children's unique needs. Limitations are imposed on many hearing conservation programs because of insufficiently high political priorities. The auditory needs of older individuals in nursing facilities are not being met, usually because professional staff in such settings are not adequately informed.

Even so, the services for the hard of hearing and deaf continue to expand and improve. Medical research and treatment procedures provide new insights into prevention and therapy. Experiences with surgical technique, hardware, and rehabilitative methods in persons having cochlear implants should have important future implications. Hearing aids reflect new developments in electroacoustic design. Newly designed amplifying systems are providing expanded listening opportunities for the hard-of-hearing in churches and theaters. Tactile and visual warning systems and telephone devices have significantly expanded the connections between deaf persons and their surrounding world. Continued research and development in these and many other areas should continue to expand future alternatives. Increased interest among hearing persons in developing manual signing skills should also facilitate this process.

SUGGESTED READINGS

For the treatment of ways in which hearing impairment and deafness are managed we recommend the following:

Bradford, L. J., and W. G. Hardy (1979). *Hearing and Hearing Impairment.* New York: Grune & Stratton. *A comprehensive treatment. It reviews medical and surgical treatment and covers each of the following topics from a variety of perspectives: educational methods and settings, special considerations for multiply handicapped children and adults, mental health and social aspects, and service delivery systems.*

Martin, F. N. (1986). *Introduction to Audiology,* 3rd ed. Englewood Cliffs, NJ: Prentice-Hall. *A popular introductory text including a review of medical and surgical treatment.*

Detailed information regarding otologic treatment and surgery may be found in any medical library. The following is one of the more recent texts.

Paparella, M. M. and D. A. Shumrick (Eds.) (1980). *Otolaryngology,* 2nd ed. Philadelphia: W. B. Saunders.

Recommended texts on the various strategies comprising audiologic management are the following:

Davis, J., and E. J. Hardick (1981). *Rehabilitative Audiology for Children and Adults.* New York: Wiley. *A broad treatment of audiologic managment.*

O'Neill, J. J., and H. J. Oyer (1981). *Visual Communication for the Hard of Hearing,* 2nd ed. Englewood Cliffs, NJ: Prentice-Hall. *This text includes more detail about speechreading.*

Pollack, M. C. (Ed.) (1987). *Amplification for the Hearing-Impaired,* 3rd ed. New York: Grune & Stratton. *A presentation of technical and applied information on hearing aids and their selection.*

The following three books are excellent introductions to historical and educational aspects of deafness.

Bender, R. E. (1970). *The Conquest of Deafness,* 2nd ed. Cleveland: Case Western Reserve Press. *A scholarly discussion of society's attitudes toward deaf persons through past centuries, covering the development of pertinent educational methods.*

Gannon, J. (1980). *Deaf Heritage: A Narrative History of Deaf America.* Silver Spring, MD: National Association of the Deaf.

Moores, D. F. (1987). *Educating the Deaf: Psychology, Principles and Practices,* 3rd ed. Boston: Houghton Mifflin. *A review of modern concepts of deaf education and counseling, including research literature in the area.*

—————————— *Study Questions* ——————————

1. Imagine that you live in the flight path of jet airplanes landing and taking off at an airport. Or that you have a new neighbor who keeps a dog in the backyard that barks every time a car passes in front of the house (including in the early morning hours). Or that you are newly employed in a shipyard and operate a gun that rivets two steel plates together; it makes so much noise that you cannot talk (or shout) with others in the area. List the comparative needs and choices you would have in each of these situations to (a) make life more tolerable, and (b) protect yourself from physical damage. In what ways do you think that governmental legislation may be helpful in these three situations?

2. You are having a conversation with a music professor over coffee. After you tell him you are studying hearing, he informs you that he has had a slowly progressive hearing loss in the higher frequencies for 30 years since he left the army, and that it has and is causing serious problems in his discipline and in class. He has never tried a hearing aid. Why do you suppose he has not done so?

3. Which of the various types of hearing aids (body, BTE, ITE, ITC) would be best to fit on a child of six months thought to have a severe hearing impairment in both ears? Why?

4. Under what circumstances do you think it would be possible for one hearing-impaired person to become a proficient speechreader whereas another person would find it an impossibly frustrating task?

5. Given the contrasts in Moores' comparative description of the normally hearing child and the profoundly deaf child (p. 207), is it realistic to expect that even in the best of educational programs the deaf child will reach the reading and writing skill level of the hearing child at age 16? Why?

6. If you were the parent of a deaf child, which of the four modes of communication discussed in this chapter would you favor as an educational method when seeking formal instruction for your child? Why? What other information, if any, would be needed before making a decision about educational placement?

10

The Profession and the Professional

The foundations of normal oral communication, and the disorders that can occur in this important human activity, have been examined throughout this text. Although reference has been made to remedial services, there obviously is more to be said about the profession of speech-language pathology and audiology itself. This chapter is about the places and the persons delivering remedial services. Throughout the descriptions of service delivery and of associated professionals, emphasis will be placed on the need for the high quality of both.

THE PROFESSION

For over 50 years there has been a helping specialty serving the communicatively disordered. At the outset, this specialty was termed "speech correction." Over the years, it has developed into a multifaceted profession, largely concerned with speech-language disorders on the one hand and hearing impairments on the other. As one might expect, within each of these two groups individual specialists have further narrowed their areas of expertise. For example, some speech-language pathologists deal primarily with persons who stutter or with adults having neurogenic disorders. Some audiologists offer primarily evaluative services while others concentrate upon rehabilitation. In the latter category are those who dispense hearing aids and provide assistance in their use.

Communication disorders specialists are employed in a great variety of settings. Their skills make them important persons in such sites and, reciprocally, such work environments further hone their skills. For example, audiologists serving persons with hearing impairments largely associated with diseases or pathologies of the ear may be found in hospitals and medical clinics as well as in otologists' offices, teaming with the medical practitioner to understand the nature of illnesses and to develop remediation plans and procedures. In the realm of speech-language pathology are those with

217

special interests and skills in children's language disorders. These specialists often work in school settings or in various preschool programs, in association with teachers and other professionals.

We shall further explore common work settings, first those serving children and then those serving adults. Keep in mind that some communication disorders specialists work in sites that serve both children and adults.

CHILDREN'S SERVICES

Children's communication disorders differ tremendously, and thus the environment in which services are provided will also vary. A child with a delay in language development might be served in a rather special center; one with a neurologic-based disorder might be treated in quite another type of setting.

A rather common service setting is in the schools, usually but not exclusively in the elementary grades. With recent changes in public laws, communication-disordered children from birth through the school-age years can be seen by school personnel. If there is some concern about language delay in a child at a very early age, that youngster might be referred to a speech-language pathologist in a school. Special education personnel in public schools may serve all children needing help, whether they are enrolled in a "public" school or not. A remedial program for a specific child might take place in another, nonpublic school or even in the child's own home.

When the disorder suggests the need for intervention, professional services are usually available in nonschool specialty programs. The nature of such "clinics" or "centers" is commonly determined by a diagnostic category, the often broad envelope encompassing a general disorder area. For example, there are specialty centers for very young children known to have neurologic disabilities, such as children with limitations in walking, in feeding themselves, in visual and hearing tasks, and in speech and language development. This group also includes youngsters whose primary problem cannot be "diagnosed," but whose secondary problems (the limitations just noted) might be responsive ("stimulable") to improvement procedures. Other specialty centers serve children who are classified as emotionally disturbed. Among the behaviors that may be observed in this group are speech and language disorders. Illustrative of this category is childhood autism. The rehabilitation team in such a center may well include a speech-language pathologist.

Although not all are exclusively for children, evaluative and remedial services are provided by hospitals to children with many types of communication disorders. Evaluation and consultation are more likely to predominate (because of transportation, fees, or other limitations on regular visits for treatment), yet remedial services are commonly offered in these sites. Speech-language pathologists in hospitals work with a large population of children with anatomic or physiologic problems. The previously noted neurogenic patient is an obvious example, but also helped are patients with congenital defects, such as cleft palate or other abnormalities associated with embryonic or fetal development. The hospital-based speech-language pathologist often acts as a "consultant" to community speech-language pathologists in more general practice. Alternatively, as mentioned above, some hospitals and medical centers provide remediation within their own walls.

Children with communication disorders are frequently enrolled in residential and custodial care centers. Speech-language pathologists and audiologists are commonly on the resident staffs of such centers, caring for the mentally retarded or emotionally disturbed youngster or children with other disorders requiring special management. Obviously, such specialists find their work highly focused. They also work with other specialized professionals in associated disciplines, including teachers, counselors, physical and occupational therapists, psychologists, nurses, and physicians.

Children with communication disorders are being served by an ever-increasing number of speech-language pathologists and audiologists in private practice. This occurs more frequently in larger cities, but in the future will undoubtedly be more available in smaller communities. Some private practitioners work in their clients' homes or in offices within their own homes. A large financial outlay is necessary for procuring the instrumentation used in audiologic practice. Yet an increasing number of audiologists are found in private practice or in association with a physician or a hospital clinic serving the hearing impaired.

ADULT SERVICES

Both speech-language pathologists and audiologists serve adults in various specialty clinics. Many rehabilitation centers assist injured adults with speech and hearing help along with physical and occupational therapy, counseling, and vocational guidance. Some speech and hearing centers (or clinics) receive financial support from community sources ("United Way"), from medical or hospital fees-for-service, or through service organizations (United Cerebral Palsy, Easter Seal, Lions, Sertoma, Scottish Rite, and others). Financial support may also derive from state and federal programs or from third-party payors (e.g., medical insurance).

As for children's communication disorders, many hospitals offer direct assistance to adults. For example, the Veterans Administration often provides speech-language pathology and audiology services to eligible persons (usually men having had military service) in their nationwide hospitals. Armed services medical centers also provide help to military personnel and their dependents (including children). Some general hospitals provide services to communicatively disordered patients, not always based upon anatomic or physiologic problems. Rehabilitation (physical) medicine and otolaryngology departments may include a component serving speech-language and/or audiology patients.

Some custodial or nursing home (long-term care) settings for geriatric patients with communication disorders also provide speech-language and hearing services, usually supported by federal and state sources. As the general population ages, this will become an even larger component of professional practice in this field. As more is known about the various conditions associated with the aging process, increasingly varied services will be offered in the area of communication disorders.

Lastly, private practitioners offer evaluative and treatment (management) services to adults as they do to children. Frequently the same practitioner serves both age groups.

TEAM PRACTICES

As is evident from the preceding discussion, speech-language pathologists and audiologists function in environments that involve other specialists—especially in hospitals, rehabilitation centers, and some small private practice groups. Many communication disorders are best approached through a team of specialists. At times, the team is "in-house," meaning that the speech-language pathologist or audiologist works in a hospital, clinic, or office that also houses the other specialists on the team. Or the team may be "ad-hoc": necessary specialists can be called upon to meet the needs of a particular patient/client; these professionals work together, perhaps not in the same building, and are "on call" when necessary.

Examples of the in-house team are the following. An audiologist may serve the patients of an otologist and may work in the same office. The otologist may need audiometric information to develop a diagnosis accurately and may refer the patient, after study, to the audiologist for rehabilitation planning. Rehabilitation may include testing for and fitting of a hearing aid or other assistive listening device. Some audiologists serve in special education departments of school systems, working together with the special education team: the nurse, psychologist, counselor, or remedial teaching specialists, for example.

Other in-house practices involve speech-language pathologists serving in hospitals. Acute-care hospitals, those serving patients with rapid onset of serious illness or injury, often have speech-language pathologists working with other specialties such as rehabilitation medicine or pediatrics. Patients having brain injuries, for example, may be hospitalized because of life-threatening conditions. As these patients recover, the "rehabilitation team" can become involved—including not only speech-language pathology specialists, but physical, occupational, or respiratory therapists; neurology specialists; vocational or other counselors; or any of a large group of other specialty-trained personnel. The function of the speech-language pathologist may be to assist the patient in rudimentary communication (perhaps through an augmentative communication device) with hospital personnel and family, in improving feeding and swallowing processes, or in redeveloping lost skills in speech and language. Such in-house teams also function in cerebral palsy rehabilitation centers, geriatric long-term care facilities, hospitals for emotionally disturbed patients, and a host of other special rehabilitation custodial-care facilities.

"Ad-hoc" teams may spring up spontaneously as the need arises. An aphasic patient, having been discharged from an acute care hospital to his/her home, may travel from home to a physical or occupational therapist or to a speech-language pathologist, while the neurologist is kept informed about the patient's progress in each treatment program. A child with a cleft lip and palate will be served by a speech-language pathologist, a plastic surgeon, an otologist and associated audiologist, a dental specialist, and others as needed. Such a team usually maintains communication among its members as they move the child progressively through an habilitation program. Other disorders may require similarly organized, "as-needed" teams of specialists to meet a particular patient's needs; the patient travels from his/her home to a particular specialist rather than to a single center where all are housed and work together.

Because of the great variety of individuals served by communication disorders specialists and the variety of such disorders, not all patients "fit" easily into all teams. Often other specialists may be called in, though perhaps not regularly. For example, most patients with cleft lip and palate are referred for consultation with a specialist in genetics. Such may not be the case for a patient with aphasia. The individual patient and his/her problems dictate the makeup of a team.

One common activity in habilitation-rehabilitation is counseling. In many cases, it is essential to inform the patient, friends, and relatives about the nature of the problem, the procedures recommended to resolve the problem, and any risks involved in such procedures. Counselors may be interpreters of information from specialists. They may be stimulators to enhance active participation of patients and family in the rehabilitation program. Counselors may explain rules and regulations (e.g., governmental or insurance funding for various rehabilitation activities). They may act to resolve negative influences in rehabilitation programs, such as family discord, financial support problems, transportation difficulties, and personal feelings and emotions that inhibit active participation. The counselor actually may be the rehabilitation specialist (e.g., the speech-language pathologist, the audiologist, or the plastic surgeon) or may be a medical social worker, a public health nurse, or an educational or other counselor.

Payment for these services can be difficult for some patients. Fees for rehabilitation can amount to hundreds of dollars per week, and entering into a contract for those services is not easily done. Guidance to third-party payors is often necessary. In some instances, the patient (or parent) has health insurance that covers audiologic and/or speech-language pathology services.

Funding for services to persons with communication disorders is often covered by governmental agencies. For example, military veterans under certain circumstances may apply to Veterans Administration hospitals for communication disorders services. Active military and certain other governmental employee groups are often served by military medical centers. Federal and state funds often assist children and adults with hearing and expressive disorders; these persons may be served through the state or county (public) health departments. Health maintenance organizations, medical programs for which enrollees pay monthly fees, may serve member-patients with communication disorders.

OTHER PROFESSIONAL ROLES

In addition to providing direct services to communicatively impaired children and adults, speech-language pathologists and audiologists may assume professional responsibilities of a different type. The following represent some that are conducted by a substantial number of professionals in the field.

Academic Teaching and Research

Important aspects of any profession are the processes of educating those who wish to practice it and pursuing new knowledge through research. The academic programs in institutions of higher education that offer instructional programs in speech-language pathology and audiology include a large number of skilled didactic and clinical teachers, as well as those conducting research into the normal and disordered aspects of human oral communication. Persons wishing for professorial appointments in colleges and universities ordinarily must complete requirements for the doctoral degree (usually Ph.D. or Ed.D.) so that they are prepared to conduct independent research as well as classroom instruction. Some educators at the doctoral level are also qualified clinicians and engage in the clinical supervision of students. A significant number of skilled clinicians with education at the master's degree level are also employed by colleges and universities for the same purpose.

Administration

Professional service and educational programs, consisting of many staff members and large budgets, must be administered by qualified individuals who provide adequate leadership in program operation and development. Many individuals in the profession move into such positions, usually after having had significant experience in the field. Administrative roles may be occupied by those at both doctoral and master's levels and can be found in all the clinical service and educational settings described above. Some professionals also assume administrative responsibilities in federal and state governmental agencies concerned with matters associated with the communication sciences and disorders.

Industrial Audiology

The problem of noise in our society, which was discussed in Chapter 9, has attracted the attention of many audiologists as a professional specialty. The focus is on the prevention of hearing impairment in populations subjected to high levels of noise. These audiologists, often in association with physicians and acoustical engineers, concentrate on the identification of potentially damaging noise sources; provision of protective devices (such as earplugs or earmuffs) to those working in such environments; monitoring the hearing status of endangered employees over time; and counseling the employer on ways in which noise might be reduced at the source, among other matters. Some of these audiologists are employed by a specific industrial concern, whereas others offer their services on a contractual basis to a number of companies. Some audiologists act as consultants to the health departments of state and urban jurisdictions regarding community noise and its prevention.

Other industrial or commercial positions held by audiologists entail research and development of hearing instruments (audiometers, aids, and assistive devices). Of course, some audiologists (appropriately licensed) sell and service hearing aids for hearing-impaired customers.

WHERE TO LOOK FOR SERVICES

An excellent source of information about the location of professional services in the United States is the national association serving specialists working and studying in the area of human communication disorders. This is the American Speech-Language-Hearing Association. Its national offices are in Rockville, Maryland, adjacent to Washington, DC (10801 Rockville Pike, MD 20852). It establishes and monitors the standards of the profession (described later). It also offers an information source for persons seeking help for a communication disorder: telephone 1-800-638-8255 during eastern-time work hours. This is always an excellent beginning.

Another information source is the nearest major university or college. It may have a training or education program for developing specialists in communication disorders. Some universities have a speech and hearing clinic or center that stands alone or one associated with a medical school or a special education department. A general information office can usually direct an inquiry to the right place.

Many major hospitals provide services for the communication-disordered person. A telephone call or letter to such a hospital, directed to the speech-language or hearing clinic, should elicit a helpful response.

Most public school programs have speech-language pathologists and audiologists serving their children. A call to the special education division or the district school superintendent's office, or even to a nearby elementary school, may stimulate action to provide help for a child with a speech-language or hearing disorder.

The yellow pages of telephone directories may have listings for specialists. On finding and contacting such an individual one may discover that the particular service being sought is not offered by that person or clinic, but this specialist may be able to guide the caller to another source of help.

Of course, in all contacts one must ensure that the person is competent and the center is approved. Methods by which individual practitioners become professionally qualified and service programs become accredited are important aspects of any profession serving the public.

STANDARDS OF THE PROFESSION

The origins of speech-language pathology and audiology as a profession can be traced back to 1925. In that year, a group of ten people concerned about disordered speech organized an association to encourage research and the exchange of information on communication disorders and to establish high standards of clinical competence in those who provide services to the public.

Concern for establishing such standards arose from evidence that many communicatively handicapped individuals were paying untrained individuals for treatment programs, many of which were "guaranteed" to produce "normal" speech behavior. Notorious examples of this were many such services advertised as a "cure" of stuttering. Schools were established in which students agreed to keep the "secrets" of their therapy from others; treatment was even provided through correspondence courses. The situation was not unlike that experienced in the early days of many other professions, such as medicine. Similar concerns were raised later about the sale of hearing aids to hearing-impaired persons. Once electronic amplifiers became wearable, they were often sold on a door-to-door basis to anyone that could be convinced that one (and sometimes two) was needed—regardless of the nature, extent, or physical cause of the hearing loss.

It is for these reasons that professions providing direct services to the public have developed basic standards of practice within the boundaries of their professional responsibilities. These standards have become the guidelines used in the education and training of those wishing to achieve recognition as competent practitioners in a profession. Further, they form the basis for evaluating the ethics and practices of those engaged in providing services to the public. These standards are often solidified into the laws and regulations of state governments as legal assurance of reasonable public protection from unprofessional conduct.

The delineation of professional standards has been a major activity of the national organization representing those working in the field, the American Speech-Language-Hearing Association. (Although the word "language" is in its title, it is still referred to as "ASHA," based on its former name: American Speech and Hearing Association.) It represents over 50,000 members, the majority engaged as clinicians offering evaluative and rehabilitative services directly to the public.

The Association's highly organized standards program operates in four major areas: (1) certification of individual practitioners; (2) accreditation of educational institutions offering programs of study at the master's level; (3) accreditation of programs providing professional services in the field; and (4) enforcement of a Code of Ethics subscribed to by its members. These programs have been of considerable assistance in promoting consistent standards of educational and service delivery in the various states. The standards associated with the first three areas above are developed by a semi-autonomous body called the Council on Professional Standards in Speech-Language Pathology and Audiology. An Ethical Practices Board monitors the ethical code and may investigate charges of unethical conduct lodged against members of the association. Let us examine each of these activities in greater detail.

Individual Certification Standards

In the early 1950s, ASHA established a voluntary program providing recognition to those who could demonstrate satisfactory completion of specified academic work and supervised clinical experience. Later, applicants were expected to pass a national written examination in the field. This voluntary program led to the award of what is now called the Certificate of Clinical Competence (CCC) in either speech-language pathology or audiology. Until recent years, when some states started licensing those working in this area, possessing the CCC was the only way in which individuals could demonstrate that they were formally recognized by their peers as competent clinicians in the profession. The certificate is generally accepted by employers and the general public as evidence that a person has the qualifications for working as an independent practitioner, especially in those states not requiring professional licensure or registration. One does not need to be a member of ASHA to apply for and receive the CCC. However, ASHA requires that those of its members who provide clinical services must be certified.

The current requirements for ASHA certification can be summarized as follows:

- Specific course content and academic credits in preprofessional and graduate courses, including the award of the master's degree or its equivalent in the field.
- Supervised clinical experience (minimum of 300 clock hours after Jan. 1, 1993 350 clock hrs. will be needed) with a variety of children and adults having communication disorders. This practicum must include both evaluation and treatment activities.
- At least nine months of successful full-time (or equivalent part-time) work in the field, following the completion of academic experience.
- Successful completion of a written examination in the appropriate area (speech-language pathology or audiology), which is administered by a national testing service.

Since the CCC represents *minimum* standards of competence for individual clinical practice, many members of ASHA have recently supported the initiation of a recognition program for those who have developed advanced skills in working with specific types of disorders or clinical techniques. Such a program is presently under study. Standards of recognition as a specialist in a highly focused subspecialty (such as stuttering or hearing aids) have been proposed to evaluate the advanced competencies of individuals who voluntarily desire such acknowledgement.

The Association also maintains an awards program recognizing members who actively participate in continuing education activities. These include attendance at national and state conventions and workshops, completing postgraduate academic work, obtaining successful results on national certification examinations, etc. The names of individuals recognized in this way, and of those holding the CCC, are published regularly by ASHA.

State Licensure

An association of professionals in speech-language pathology and audiology exists in each of the states. These organizations provide educational activities, maintain ethical standards for their members, and deal with professional issues unique to each state jurisdiction. One active area in which many of them have been engaged has been the passage of legislation establishing licensure or registration acts in speech-language pathology and audiology. This legislation provides legal definitions of the profession, educational and experiential requirements, and acceptable modes of professional practice. Penalties for unlawful or unethical conduct have the force of law behind them. As in medicine, law, and many other professions, such laws protect the public from incompetent practices. Legislation of this type was enacted in 36 states by 1988. Most of these statutes require educational and experiential backgrounds similar to those incorporated in ASHA's CCC standards. Professional organizations with similar goals and functions serve in a number of other countries, some associated with the International Logopedia Association ("logopedia" refers to correction of speech).

Educational Standards

As stated above, ASHA has established the master's degree as the minimum level of educational preparation for those wanting recognition as competent clinicians in the field. This action was taken over 20 years ago after a national conference at which it was concluded that a four-year baccalaureate program could not provide an adequate liberal education, prerequisite coursework in the normal communication sciences, and sufficient clinical knowledge and practicum to ensure competence as an independent practitioner. Careful consideration of the minimum educational needs required led to the specification that at least 60 semester hours of relevant academic credit and laboratory experience must be obtained, half of which must relate to courses accepted for graduate credit.

Having made that decision, the Association then established a mechanism by which academic institutions could be evaluated (if they wished) to determine whether they conformed to minimum educational standards derived by the profession. The primary purpose of this program was to provide guidelines of professional preparation that could be applied throughout the country. In addition, the recognition of academic programs showing evidence of having met these standards is information helpful to prospective graduate students in their educational planning.

This work is conducted by the Educational Standards Board of the Association. ASHA's educational standards program has been recognized by the U.S. Department of Education and by the Council on Postsecondary Accreditation. Academic programs seeking accreditation are site-visited periodically to determine the adequacy of physical facilities and equipment, faculty and staff, clinical service settings for student practicum, and other matters. In early 1989, there were approximately 260 academic programs in the United States and Canada offering a master's degree in speech-language pathology and/or audiology. Of these, 171 were accredited by ASHA in one or both areas. The Association prints a list of accredited institutions in its journal ASHA. It also publishes a complete description of institutional resources and entrance requirements in these accredited programs.

Professional Service Standards

The Association recognized, also in the mid-1960s, that it could be helpful to the public (and to clinical programs) by offering a second accreditation program, one designed to recognize organizations and institutions meeting acceptable standards of professional services. This activity, conducted by the Professional Services Board of the Association, also provides periodic site visits to ensure that appropriate facilities, personnel, and clinical practices are available within an administrative structure of two or more clinicians. Over 275 programs have achieved such recognition in speech-language pathology, in audiology, or in both areas. These programs represent the service environments described earlier in this chapter. Again, ASHA periodically provides information about these service providers through its publications and public hot-line telephone service.

Ethical Standards

An important aspect of the profession's attempt to maintain a high degree of quality in the practices of those providing services is embodied in its ethical standards. All members of the association agree to abide by these standards of conduct in their professional activities. Suspected violations of the standards are investigated by the Ethical Practice Board, which can recommend that members be publicly expelled if found to be in violation of the Code of Ethics. Similar bodies exist in most state associations to ensure conformity of their members with professional standards of conduct.

The code itself is composed of six principles, including specific examples of acceptable and proscribed conduct under each. These principles encompass the following standards of conduct that should be applied by all qualified professionals in their work with the communicatively impaired:

- Individuals shall hold paramount the welfare of persons served professionally.
- Individuals shall maintain high standards of professional competence.
- Individuals' statements to persons served professionally and to the public shall provide accurate information about the nature and management of communicative disorders and about the profession and services rendered by its practitioners.
- Individuals shall maintain objectivity in all matters concerning the welfare of persons served professionally.
- Individuals shall honor their responsibilities to the public, their profession, and their relationships with colleagues and members of allied professions.
- Individuals shall uphold the dignity of the profession and freely accept the profession's self-imposed standards.

These principles are certainly not unique to the profession of speech-language pathology and audiology. In one form or another, they form the basis of all modern concepts of conduct and behavior that the public should observe in anyone providing specialized services to impaired, handicapped, or disabled adults or children. They represent the minimum expectations of both the public and the profession itself.

SUMMARY

The distinctive feature of the profession of speech-language pathology and audiology is its focus on improving oral communication in those persons with disordered speech, language, or hearing. It is a "helping" profession, composed of men and women with a variety of skills and knowledge who provide services to others in many work settings.

As in all helping professions, standards of education and training have been established to ensure the competency of those who provide their services to the public.

Similarly, standards of ethics and of professional practice delineate guidelines of quality in service delivery. These functions are important activities of the national organization representing members of the profession, the American Speech-Language-Hearing Association (ASHA).

ASHA, through its representative professional membership, has set the requirements for the Certificate of Clinical Competence in Speech-Language Pathology or Audiology. A master's degree is required, with specified didactic and laboratory experiences. Many states demand a similar level of educational preparation to earn licensure to practice in the field. This minimal level of preparation is expanded by further (post-master's degree) experience and continuing education. As a result, the practicing clinician may become specialized in specific disorders, age groupings, and clinical practice approaches.

Some individuals study toward and earn a doctoral (Ph.D.) degree. They may then pursue professional activities in teaching, research, or administration, as well as continuing to provide clinical services to the communicatively impaired. Clinical research is not restricted to doctoral level professionals, but these individuals often are in better positions (e.g., university settings) to study and produce new and improved evaluative and treatment approaches.

At the outset of this book, in Chapter 1, we reviewed the reasons why people talk to people and why this is such a unique and critically important process for human beings. Our discussion throughout the text has laid the groundwork for understanding why disorders of communication can be truly handicapping conditions and can prevent persons from reaching their full potentials and expectations as members of our human society. Those who devote their lives to the improvement of others' communication skills must demonstrate, by the extent of their education and the quality of their professional services, that they meet and surpass the standards established by their peers. These standards equally earn the trust of the clients whom they serve. Speech-language pathologists and audiologists work to develop behavioral changes in those who seek help—changes that lead to improvements in effective listening, in the conversion of thoughts and ideas into symbols, and in oral expression, in ways that positively influence other people in our surrounding world. In our lives, there is no act more human.

Appendix
Organizations Offering Further Information

Alexander Graham Bell Association for the Deaf, 3417 Volta Place NW, Washington, DC 20007. Emphasizes development of oral speech skills in hearing-impaired persons. Operates an Oral Deaf Adults Section, the International Parents Organization, and the International Organization for the Hearing Impaired. Publishes a monthly journal called *Volta Review.*

American Academy of Otolaryngology—Head and Neck Surgery, Inc., 1101 Vermont Avenue NW, Suite 302, Washington, DC 20005. Professional organization for medical specialists in otology and laryngology.

American Speech-Language-Hearing Association, 10801 Rockville Pike, Rockville, MD 20852. Professional organization for audiologists and speech-language pathologists. Certifies the clinical competence of individuals and accredits university education programs and service agencies in both fields. Publishes various journals and establishes professional standards. Provides directory of speech and hearing associations in each state.

Better Hearing Institute, 14309 K Street, NW, Suite 700, Washington, Dc 20005. Supported by major manufacturers of hearing instruments, including hearing aids, audiometers, etc. Provides consumer information.

National Association of the Deaf, 814 Thayer Avenue, Silver Spring, MD 20910. Provides information on all aspects of deafness. Common address for a number of national organizations with specific interests: **American Deafness and Rehabilitation Association; American Society for Deaf Children** (provides state listings of summer camp programs for deaf children); **Associations for Education of the Deaf; Registry of Interpreters for the Deaf;** and **Telecommunications for the Deaf, Inc.** The National Association can provide names and addresses of the various state associations for deaf individuals. The *American Annals of the Deaf* provides an annual directory of services for deaf persons.

National Hearing Aid Society, 20361 Middlebelt Road, Livonia, MI 48152. Organization for hearing-aid dispensers. Provides a voluntary certification program by correspondence and sponsors continuing education activities for dispensers.

National Information Center on Deafness, Gallaudet University, 800 Florida Avenue NE, Washington, DC 20002. Provides information on vocational training, education, technology, and other matters related to deafness, including referrals to local services.

Self-Help for Hard of Hearing People, Inc., 7800 Wisconsin Avenue, Bethesda, MD 20814. Provides information about hearing impairment, with special focus on acquired hearing loss in adults. Publishes a bimonthly journal (*SHHH*) and encourages development of local and state chapters.

The following organizations provide information about the communication disorders related to specific conditions, as usually designated in their names:

American Association of Mental Retardation,   1719 Kalorama Road NW, Washington, DC 20009.

Association for Children and Adults with Learning Disabilities,   4156 Library Road, Pittsburgh, PA 15234.

National Aphasia Association,   400 East 34th Street, New York, NY 10016.

National Council on Stuttering,   Box 8171, Grand Rapids, MI 59418.

National Head Injury Foundation,   18A Vernon Street, Framingham, MA 01701.

Orton Dyslexia Society,   724 York Road, Baltimore, MD 21204.

Speech Foundation of America,   5139 Lingle Street NW, Washington, DC 20016.
Publishes monographs on stuttering from time to time, written by experts in the field.

Glossary

Brief definitions are provided here. A comprehensive source of nomenclature used in speech-language pathology and audiology is Nicolosi, L., E. Harryman, and J. Kresheck (1989). Terminology of Communication Disorders, 3rd ed. Baltimore: Williams & Wilkins.

Abnormality: a departure from normal form or function.

Acoustic reflex: *see* Auditory reflex.

Acoustics: science of sound.

Addition: an error in articulation in which an extra phoneme is placed in a word. When this occurs because of regional dialect, it may not be considered a disorder.

Adenoid: lymphoid tissue located in the posterior wall of the nasopharynx; also known as pharyngeal tonsils.

Affective-social dimension: the support and stimulation by persons in the social environment of the child learning language and speech.

Afferent (sensory) neurons: neurons of the central nervous system that carry stimuli toward a central organ or area.

Affricate: a consonant sound that has both a fricative and stop component; for example, /ch/ in the word "church."

Agraphia: difficulties in writing.

Air conduction (AC) pathway: the route through the ear normally used by airborne sound. This pathway incorporates the entire peripheral ear and central auditory nervous system.

Alexia: difficulties in reading.

Alveolar ridge (process): crescent-shaped bony structure that houses dentition.

AM system: amplification system in which frequent fluctuations are made by alterations in amplitude in a continuous-frequency carrier.

American manual alphabet (fingerspelling): a code system, executed with one hand, that provides a specific symbol for each letter of the English alphabet.

American Sign Language (ASL): the primary visual-gestural language system of signing deaf persons in the United States. An independent language with its own vocabulary and grammatical system.

Ankyloglossia (tongue-tie): abnormal restriction of tongue-tip elevation during speech due to the presence of a membrane (frenum) between the tongue-tip and mouth floor.

Anomaly: extreme variation from normal, usually in reference to anatomy.

Anomia: "nominal" or "semantic" aphasia; a type of fluent aphasia in which the person is unable to find a word or name for which he/she is searching.

ANSI: American National Standards Institute: organization that sets physical standards, e.g., sound pressure levels representing normal hearing thresholds.

Aphasia: disorders in the use of language usually stemming from injury to the left hemisphere of the brain.

Aphonia: a complete lack of laryngeal tone; voicelessness.

Apraxia: a disturbance in normal volitional muscle movement patterns due to left cerebral hemisphere damage.

Articulation: production of speech sounds, especially the vowels and consonants.

Articulation disorder: a problem in speech-sound (phoneme) production that attracts negative attention or lessens intelligibility and/or disturbs the speaker.

Articulators: anatomic structures that manipulate the airstream in speech (mandible, tongue, lips, teeth, alveolar ridge, hard and soft palate).

ASHA: American Speech-Language-Hearing Association, the national professional society of scholars and clinicians interested in normal and disordered communication processes.

Aspiration: intake of foreign material into the lungs during the act of breathing or swallowing.

Audibility: the capacity to hear sound.

Audiogram: a chart for recording the frequency and intensity of auditory thresholds obtained for pure tones.

Audiologist: a specialist in evaluating auditory function, in the conservation of hearing, and in the nonmedical management of hearing impairment.

Audiology: the field and profession concerned with the evaluation and conservation of hearing function and the amelioration of disordered hearing in medically irreversible auditory impairment.

Audio loop system: a sound transmission system that uses inductance on an individual receiver in a magnetic field to transmit an audio signal to listeners within that field.

Audiometer: an instrument used in determining hearing sensitivity and other aspects of hearing function.

Audition: the process of hearing.

Auditory feedback: monitoring one's own vocalization through hearing.

Auditory monitoring theory: the notion that stutterers' audible perception of their own speech is quite different from that of nonstutterers.

Auditory nerve: the portion of cranial nerve VIII connecting the cochlea to the brainstem; also called the cochlear nerve.

Auditory perception: identification and interpretation of sensory data received through the ear.

Auditory reflex: involuntary contraction of middle-ear muscles (usually the stapedius) in response to loud sound.

Auditory school: a unisensory approach to aural rehabilitation supporting oral speech expression and strongly emphasizing auditory over visual recognition skills as the primary receptive mode. Speechreading, writing, and reading take a secondary role to the development of listening skills.

Auditory training: educational techniques designed to enhance auditory recognition of environmental sounds and speech.

Auditory (Eustachian) tube: an opening between the pharynx and middle ear providing ventilation to maintain a balance of air pressure between the middle and external ear and drainage of the middle ear when mucus or other fluids form.

Augmentative communication: the use of nonvocal instruments and approaches by those who cannot communicate vocally; includes picture boards and computer-assisted devices.

Auricle (pinna):   cartilaginous structure at the opening to the ear canal.

Autism: extreme self-absorption in thought and behavior.

Autonomic nervous system: a portion of the nervous system that acts without the conscious control of the individual; controlling, for example, the glandular system.

Avoidance phase: the efforts made by the stuttering child to avoid stuttering.

Back vowel: vowel sound produced by the arching or adjustment of the tongue in the back part of the mouth.

Basilar membrane: membrane separating the scala media from the scala tympani in the cochlea. The sensory end organ of hearing (organ of Corti) lies on this membrane.

Benign: denoting a condition capable of disturbing the structure or function of an organ; not malignant.

Bifid: divided into two parts.

Binaural: involving the use of both ears.

Biofeedback therapy: a means of teaching patients how to monitor their own speech activities and compare them with a standard.

Bolus: food that has been masticated and mixed with saliva and mucus; passes into and through the digestive tract.

Bone-conduction oscillator: a vibrator, usually attached to a hearing aid, that transmits sound to the cochlea through the skull.

Bone conduction (BC) pathway: the route by which sound enters the cochlea through the skull, primarily bypassing the outer and middle ears. Sound intensity must be reasonably high and closely coupled to the head for hearing to occur.

Bound morpheme: a language element that carries specific meaning, but cannot be uttered meaningfully by itself; for example, the plural /s/ in "cats."

Brain: that part of the central nervous system contained in the cranial cavity, consisting of the cerebrum, cerebellum, midbrain, pons, and medulla oblongata.

Brainstem: the portion of the brain consisting of midbrain, pons, and medulla oblongata.

Breathiness: the presence of audible airflow through the larynx during speech.

Broca's area: the motor speech area or speech-programming region in the cerebral cortex.

Bronchi: primary ventilation divisions of the trachea which divide to penetrate the lungs, one for the right lung and the other for the left lung.

Central deficit: a category of impaired auditory function resulting from a disorder within the central auditory nervous system.

Central nervous system: neurologic areas housed within the bones of the cranium and the vertebrae that receive, transmit, and store neurologic information; the brain and the spinal cord.

Cerebral cortex: "gray" matter covering the two cerebrums of the brain, containing major centers for receiving and sending neural impulses.

Cerebral dominance theory: in stuttering, the notion that a lack of dominance of one cerebral hemisphere leads to confusion in the speech apparatus.

Cerebral palsy: a brain injury causing any impairment of neurologic function, dating from birth or early infancy, usually without clinical evidence of progression, and generally characterized by obvious motor deficits.

Cerebrum: largest and uppermost portions of the brain (hemispheres) containing center, pathways, and (cerebral) cortex.

Certification: a statement by an officially recognized and legally constituted body that a person or institution has met or complied with certain standards of professional education or practice.

Cerumen: ear wax produced in the ear canal.

Cilia: hairlike structures at the surface of sensory cells.

Circumlocution: a roundabout way of speaking; avoiding a spoken expression.

Cleft lip: a split or opening in the upper lip, occurring if the lip fails to fuse early in embryonic development.

Cleft palate: an anatomic growth failure occurring during embryonic development, causing the nasal cavity to be connected to the oral cavity through the unfused bony or soft palate.

Cochlea: space within the temporal bone occupied by the sensory portion of the inner ear, shaped like a snail shell. It is divided into the scala vestibuli and the scala tympani (containing perilymph) and the scala media (containing endolymph and the organ of Corti).

Cochlear implant: electromagnetic device designed to stimulate sensory components remaining in the cochlea of persons with severe or profound hearing impairment who cannot use hearing aids effectively. The unit is surgically implanted into the ear.

Cognition: *see* Intellectual capacity, Intelligence.

Communication: the act of conveying or imparting information or knowledge.

Communication disorder: an observed disturbance in the normal processes of speech, language, or hearing.

Compression wave: a progressive expansion of compressed molecules in a medium, continuously moving in the direction of original displacement.

Conduction aphasia: an aphasia due to a disruption in the pathway between Wernicke's area (language formulation) and Broca's area (motor speech programming).

Conductive hearing impairment: reduced audibility due to dysfunction of the conductive system.

Conductive system: the major mechanical role played by the outer and middle ears in providing an efficient pathway for sound to enter the cochlea.

Congenital: existing before or at birth.

Consonants: phonemes whose articulation requires vocal-tract constriction creating audible airflow and pressure events.

Content: word meaning or semantics.

Contralateral: opposite; acting in concert with a similar part on the opposite side of the body.

Core behaviors: primary speech interruptions associated with stuttering that include repetitions, prolongations, pauses, and hesitations.

Cortex: the external layer of a structure, such as the cerebral cortex or the cerebellar cortex.

Cranial nerves: twelve pairs of nerves responsible for both motor and sensory functions, entering the brain with sensory information and leaving the brain with motor commands.

Deaf: a condition of severe to profound reduction in binaural audibility, resulting in minimal effective use of the auditory channel in interhuman communication even under ideal sound-amplifying conditions. The primary receptive channel is visual.

Decibel (dB): unit of sound intensity (logarithmic ratio of one sound intensity to another).

Deficiency: a lack of some necessary quality.

Degeneration: a gradual decrease of the ability of an organ, muscle, or nerve to function.

Deglutition: swallowing.

Diagnosogenic: in a theory of the origin of stuttering, caused by the child having been labeled a stutterer, with the child learning and behaving under negative communication influences.

Diphthongs: the blending of two vowels.

Disability: the limitation of normal behaviors, e.g., gainful employment, because of a physical or functional impairment.

Discrimination score: percentage of words correctly identified from a list of monosyllabic words presented at a comfortable loudness.

Disfluency: any type of speech that is marked with repetitions, prolongations, and hesitations; an interruption in the flow of speech-sounds; stuttering.

Disorder: extreme variation from the normal function; in speech or hearing, leading to observable characteristics, lowered communicative intelligibility, and/or self-image (personal) concepts deleterious to the speaker or listener.

Dissonance: sound occurring when the frequencies of a stimulus are not in harmonic relationship.

Distortion: articulation errors that cause the intended phoneme to be heard as something other than the intended sound, yet not as another speech sound of the language.

Dorsum: upper surface, such as the large upper surface of the tongue.

Dysarthria: a neuromotor speech disorder, possibly disturbing phonation, resonance, and/or articulation.

Dysfunction: abnormality or impairment of function.

Dysphagia: swallowing disorders.

Dysphonia: a problem of voice initiated at the vocal folds; phonatory disorder.

Ear canal (external auditory meatus): opening in the temporal bone between the auricle and the tympanic membrane. It provides a protective environment for the tympanic membrane, ensuring that the temperature and humidity in the immediate area remain reasonably constant.

Eardrum: *see* Tympanic membrane.

Echolalia: vocal repetition of what one hears.

Edentulous: toothless.

Efferent (motor) neurons: motor nerve fibers leaving the central nervous system nuclei via the cranial or spinal nerves.

Effusion: fluid accumulated in the middle ear, usually accompanying otitis media.

Electronystagmography: a test of vestibular function, involving the recording of muscular movements around the eyes in response to stimulation of the vestibular system.

Embryo: the first period (in humans the first two months) of developing life after conception.

Endolymph: one of the two fluids found in the cochlea (scala media) and vestibular system.

End organ: the termination of nerve fibers in muscle, skin, or other structure, e.g., organ of Corti in the cochlea.

Epiglottis: a pharyngeal structure that partially covers the entrance to the larynx.

Esophageal speech: technique to develop a new source of phonation (e.g., following laryngectomy) whereby air injected into the esophagus is used to vibrate tissues to create sound.

Esophagus: the portion of the digestive canal between the pharynx and stomach.

Ethics: principles of proper conduct: the set of moral values, as well as professionally endorsed principles and practices, that govern the conduct of a member of a profession in its exercise.

Etiology: the cause (or causes) of a disorder or impairment.

Eustachian (auditory) tube: *see* Auditory tube.

Evoked response audiometry: recording of electrical activity within the auditory system as it is stimulated by certain sounds.

Expressive aphasia: difficulties in forming and uttering language.

Expressive language: communication through the spoken or printed word, or other forms.

External auditory meatus: *see* Ear canal.

Facial paralysis: paralysis of the muscles of the face, which occurs if the facial nerve (VII) is damaged.

Falsetto: higher regions of pitch range in normal phonation, at times used to such an extent as to be considered a phonatory disorder.

Feature: a prominent characteristic in articulation used to describe a phoneme: place, manner, and voicing.

Fistula: an abnormal opening into a cavity.

Fluency: the forward flow of speech with lack of hesitations or repetitions in speaking.

FM system: amplification system in which the frequency of a continuous-amplitude carrier wave is varied by the audio input.

Form: the accepted sequence for meaningful utterances of phonemes and words; grammar or syntax.

Free morpheme: an element of language that carries meaning when standing alone, e.g., "cat."

Frenum: thin fold of mucous membrane interconnecting the undersurface of the tongue-tip and the floor of the mouth, or the lips and the alveolar ridges; either may be abnormally extensive and restrictive.

Frequency of sound: the vibratory rate of a sound-producing object in a medium, measured in Hertz; the number of complete periods of condensations and rarefactions occurring each second.

Fricative: a consonant produced when flowing, pressurized air is forced through the constriction of articulators.

Frontal lobe: anterior section of the brain which serves as the primary motor area to the body's muscular system, as well as providing for memory, cognition, and personality functions.

Fundamental frequency: lowest component frequency of a periodic wave.

Ganglion: an accumulation of nerve cell bodies.

Genetics: the science that deals with hereditary characteristics transmitted by genes.

Geriatric: pertaining to the process of aging.

Gingiva: the mucosa covering the alveolar ridge and palate; "gums."

Glides: consonants produced by articulatory movement toward or away from constriction; as in /w/, /j/, /r/, and sometimes /hw/.

Glossectomy: surgical removal of a portion of the entire tongue, usually for the prevention of the spread of cancer.

Glossopharyngeal ("frog") breathing: a breathing technique in which the patient learns to pump small bubbles of air into the airway in a gulping fashion, which can then be maneuvered into the lungs. It is used as a safeguard system for patients who need rudimentary breathing techniques for respiratory paralysis.

Glottal: a fricative produced by aerodynamic turbulence at the vocal folds, as in /h/ or a glottal stop.

Glottis: the space between the vocal folds.

Habitual pitch level: the easiest or most natural pitch level for a person to use.

Hair cell: a specialized sensory structure of the cochlea and vestibular system that must be stimulated to obtain auditory or balance sensations.

Handicap: difficulty in achieving normal expectations in daily living due to an impairment.

Hard-of-hearing: having a partial hearing impairment in which the auditory system is the primary receptive channel, with or without amplification.

Hard (bony) palate: anterior part of the roof of the mouth.

Harmonics: integral multiples of a sound's fundamental frequency, with the fundamental frequency being the first harmonic; the second harmonic is also called the first overtone.

Harshness: a type of dysphonia in which the laryngeal tone is irregular, sometimes in combination with hard glottal attack.

Hearing aid: any device worn by a listener to improve sound perception; typically a miniature electronic amplifier worn at one or both ears.

Hearing disorder/impairment: abnormal auditory function usually resulting in reduced auditory sensitivity and/or speech recognition.

Hearing level (HL): decibels above the normal hearing threshold level (ANSI) for a specified sound.

Hearing screening test: a simple test of hearing sensitivity designed to identify individuals who may need more careful evaluation or medical attention.

Hereditary: genetically transmitted from parent to offspring.

Hertz (Hz): unit of sound frequency (number of vibrations each second).

High vowel: vowel sound produced when the tongue is high in the mouth.

Hoarseness: a type of dysphonia, usually the result of changes in vocal folds due to vocal abuse. It is heard as a combination of breathiness with hard glottal attack or as forcefulness in vibration.

Homophonous: a descriptor of words having the same general appearance on the lips, such as "mud" and "mutt."

Hypernasality: a resonance problem created by abnormal coupling of nasal chambers to the oral cavity; may be heard in the voices of persons with cleft palate or paralyzed palate musculature.

Hypoglossal nerve: cranial nerve XII, carrying motor stimuli to the tongue and strap muscles.

Hyponasality: too little nasal quality in speech, as when one has a bad cold.

Hypoxia: lack of oxygen.

Immittance audiometry: test of middle-ear function that measures the relative impedance to the passage of a sound signal at the eardrum.

Impairment: reduced function.

Impedance: degree of opposition to the flow of energy.

Incus: one of the three bones (ossicles) in the middle ear; connects the malleus and the stapes.

Individualized Education Plan: an annually updated plan for the education of handicapped children, prepared in the educational environment and approved by the parents.

Infection: the invasion of a host by organisms, with resulting undesirable effects.

Inflammation: a local response to tissue injury that is marked by swelling, pain, and redness.

Inner ear: the part of the ear comprising the cochlear end organ, auditory nerve, and central auditory nervous system.

Intellectual capacity: the ability of a child or adult to learn; intelligence or cognition is exemplified by the ability to identify objects and events, to understand, differentiate, learn, and perceive.

Intelligence: the capacity to acquire and apply knowledge.

Intelligibility: level of being understood or comprehended.

Intensity of sound: a sound's force, energy, or pressure, measured in decibels.

Intermittency: occasions of phonatory cessation at inappropriate moments while talking.

International Phonetic Alphabet: the international standard symbol system serving to transcribe the speech (vowels, consonants, prosody, and unique sound productions) of speakers of all languages.

Intonation: the rise and fall in pitch of the voice in speech.

Labyrinth: in hearing, the space in the temporal bone consisting of the cochlea, vestibule, and the semicircular canals.

Language: " . . . a code whereby ideas about the world are represented through a conventional system of arbitrary signals for communication." (Bloom, L., and M. Lahey (1978). *Language Development and Language Disorders.* New York: John Wiley & Sons).

Language disorder: a problem involving the linguistic aspects of oral communication. Meaning, communicative intent, and linguistic code of the utterance may not be conveyed successfully.

Laryngeal tone: a sound initiated at the vocal folds.

Laryngectomy: surgical removal of the larynx due to life-endangering pathology within the larynx.

Laryngopharynx: the lowest portion of the pharynx into which air and sound enter from the larynx; hypopharynx.

Larynx: valvular structure of the airway between pharynx and trachea, acting to protect the lungs from invasion of foreign matter and serving as the primary means of generating vocal tone in speech (phonation).

Lateral lisp: an articulation disorder involving direct airflow over one or both sides of the tongue-tip, not over the end.

Laterals: consonants involving constriction by the sides of the tongue, as in the liquids (/l/ and /r/).

Levator palatine muscle: the primary muscle of the velum, contracting to elevate the velum in velopharyngeal closure, during deglutition and speaking.

Linguistic capacity: a "potential" for language processing and learning.

Linguistics: the study of language.

Lisping: disordered /s/-type sound produced by unusual constrictions and airflow with audible turbulence, quite different from the intended /s/.

Loudness: the perceptual function associated primarily with the amount of intensity information arriving at the auditory cortex.

Lymphoid tissue: the palatine, pharyngeal, and lingual tonsils usually found in the vocal tract during childhood.

Malformation: a defect or deformity.

Malignant: denoting any disease resistant to treatment and having a potentially fatal result.

Malleus: one of the three ossicles in the middle ear, attached directly to the tympanic membrane.

Malocclusion: misalignment between upper and lower teeth.

Manner: one of the features in articulation describing the acoustic or auditory nature of the phoneme (e.g., stop or fricative).

Manual signing: method of communication that utilizes a rapid succession of specific gestures, including fingerspelling.

Masking: in audiometry, the use of a sound stimulus in the nontest ear to prevent its perception of a signal in the test ear.

Mastication: chewing, pulverizing of food.

Mean length of utterance (MLU): the average number of words or morphemes an individual uses in a talking event.

Memory: the faculty of the mind by which ideas and sensations are recalled.

Meniere's disease: a condition associated with the production of excessive endolymphatic fluid in the cochlea and connecting labyrinth. Its symptoms include the sudden occurrence of severe dizziness and nausea, accompanied by hearing loss and tinnitus.

Meningitis: inflammation of the membranes covering the brain or spinal cord.

Metabolic disorders: impairments caused by abnormal chemical changes in the body processes.

Metalinguistic: having personal knowledge of language itself, e.g., knowing that a word is symbolic.

Middle ear: the air-filled cavity between the outer and inner ears that contains the tympanic ossicles, muscles, and ligaments.

Mixed hearing impairment: reduced auditory function comprising both conductive and sensorineural impairments.

Monaural: involving the use of one ear.

Monopitch/monotone: voice production in speech with little or no pitch variation.

Morpheme: smallest unit of spoken language carrying specific meaning.

Morphology: study of language structure, including phonology and syntax, i.e., the rules for the use of phonemes and for grammar in a language.

Motor nerve: *see* Efferent neurons.

Multiple sclerosis: a condition in which the myelin sheath of nerves provides insufficient insulation, resulting in impaired neural functioning.

Myasthenia gravis: a neuromuscular disease characterized by abnormal muscular fatigability.

Myelin sheath: the insulating cover surrounding the fibers of certain nerves.

Myringotomy: a surgical procedure in which a small incision is made in the tympanic membrane. This must be done when placing a pressure-equalizing tube in the tympanic membrane for treatment of otitis media.

Nasal consonants: in English, three phonemes normally produced by coupling the nasal and oral cavities; the /m/, /n/, and /ng/ sounds.

Nasal pharynx: the uppermost region of the pharynx serving the respiratory function, biologically, and adding nasal resonance to the voice; nasopharynx.

Nasal resonance: energy pattern added to the spectrum of a speech sound when the nasal tract is coupled to the vocal tract.

Nasal septum: the "wall" between the two chambers of the nose. It is both cartilaginous and bony in nature.

Neoplasm: literally "new tissue," as in abnormal growths such as tumors, polyps, and nodules.

Nerve pathways: tracts of nerve fibers passing from one nucleus or center to another.

Neuroglia: the supporting and protective material for the neurons in both the brain and spinal cord.

Neuron: a nerve cell body and its processes (axon and dendrites) which carry nerve impulses.

Nodule/node: in laryngeal pathology associated with phonatory disorder, a small circumscribed abnormal growth or swelling on the margin of the vocal fold.

Nonverbal: involving minimal or no use of language.

Normal hearing: average pure-tone and speech thresholds of young, otologically normal listeners.

Normal nonfluency: the speech of a child that occasionally may be hesitant and repetitive, suggesting stuttering.

Nuclei: nerve centers receiving messages from the body and sending commands to the peripheral body parts; provide interconnecting centers within the central nervous system.

Object permanence: perceptual acknowledgment of an object's existence when it is not visible; e.g., a child's searching for a hidden toy.

Occipital lobe: the back or posterior portion of the brain's cerebral cortex, largely serving the sensations of vision.

Occult (hidden) cleft palate: a form of cleft palate in which the palatal shelves fail to fuse. However, the mucous membranes that line the oral cavity cover the unfused bone; "submucous cleft palate."

Olfaction: the sense of smell.

Omission: an articulation error in which the speech-sound required in a word is not uttered.

Optimum pitch level: the "natural pitch" of voice; in the normal speaker this should be similar to habitual pitch.

Oral approach: the position that natural language learning and speech expression is so much a part of "normal" functioning in society that it should be the only acceptable communicative avenue used in educating hearing-impaired individuals.

Oral cavity/oral cavity proper: that part of the mouth chamber within the dental arches and in front of the entrance to the pharynx.

Oral pharynx: the middle pharyngeal chamber that serves both the digestive and respiratory functions, as well as providing vocal resonance; oropharynx.

Organ of Corti: a specialized receptor organ in the cochlea designed to activate the auditory nerve in response to sound stimulation.

Ossicles: the malleus, incus, and stapes bones that form the bridge across the middle ear space; ossicular chain.

Otitis media: an abnormal condition of the middle ear due to poor function of the auditory tube, infection, and/or the results of disease.

Otolaryngologist: a physician specializing in care of the ear, nose, and throat.

Otologist: a physician specializing in care of the ear.

Otosclerosis: an abnormal growth of bony tissue usually occurring at the base of the stapes in the oval window, typically causing a conductive hearing loss.

Ototoxic: causing damage to the auditory and/or vestibular system, usually due to ingestion of certain drugs.

Outer (external) ear: most peripheral portion of the ear, comprising the auricle and external ear canal.

Oval window: an opening in the temporal bone leading to the vestibule and scala vestibuli in the cochlea; contains the footplate of the stapes.

Overtone: integral multiple of a sound's fundamental frequency, with the first overtone being the second harmonic.

Palate: roof of the mouth; includes the anterior portion (hard palate) and the posterior portion (soft palate or velum).

Paralysis: loss of voluntary muscular function.

Parietal lobe: the upper back portion of the brain's cerebral cortex, largely serving body sensations (e.g., touch, heat, pressure).

Pathology: the anatomic and physiologic deviations from the normal that constitute disease or malfunction.

Perception: recognition in response to sensory stimuli; the mental act or process by which the memory or certain qualities of an act, experience, or object are associated with other qualities impressing the senses, thereby making possible recognition and interpretation of the new sensory data.

Perilymph: one of the two fluids in the cochlea (scala vestibuli and scala tympani) and the vestibular system.

Peripheral nervous system: organized nerves carrying afferent impulses (i.e., sensations) into the central nervous system and carrying efferent (i.e., motor) impulses to muscles and glands.

Peristalsis: a mostly involuntary muscular contraction throughout the entire digestive tract, carrying the bolus (of food) through the system for nutritional extraction.

Perseveration: a general type of behavioral disorder in which the person has the tendency to continue performing an act beyond its appropriateness.

Pharynx: the musculomembranous tube situated at the back of the nose, mouth, and larynx and extending from the base of the skull to a point level with the lower larynx; it becomes continuous with the esophagus. It serves vocal resonance, respiratory, and digestive systems.

Phonation: sound resulting from vocal fold vibration in a pressurized flow of air for voice production in speech.

Phonemes: a closely related group of speech-sounds or phones, represented by a single symbol in the International Phonetic Alphabet.

Phonetics: the study of speech sounds and prosody.

Phonology: the rules and customs of phoneme use in a particular language.

Pinna: *see* Auricle.

Pitch: the perceptual function associated primarily with the amount of frequency information arriving at the auditory cortex.

Pitch level: the perceptual tonal level, corresponding to frequency of a voice.

Pitch range: the available vocal tones from low to high, covering about two octaves in the normal voice.

Place: one of the features in articulation describing the anatomic location of constriction in the vocal tract (commonly the oral cavity proper), contributing to the creation of the acoustic event identified as a consonant; e.g., linguadental.

Polyp: abnormal soft tissue neoplasm; when found in the larynx can create airway threats or phonation impedances.

Pragmatics: the meaningful order in a particular situation, environment, or social context in which the speaker uses semantic and syntactic dimensions to convey meaning.

Prelingual deafness: hearing impairment occurring before the development of speech and language.

Presbycusis/presbyacusis: impaired hearing associated with aging.

Pressure-equalizing tubes: small plastic tubes surgically placed (temporarily) in the tympanic membrane for the treatment of otitis media, serving to equalize air pressure in the external and middle ear.

Prosody: acoustic/auditory character of speech as indicated by melody or inflection, involving the combination of frequency (pitch), intensity (loudness), resonance (quality), and duration at both the word and sentence levels.

Prosthesis: a device to supplement or replace a damaged or missing part of the body.

Prosthodontist: a dental specialist who fabricates dentures and other prosthetic appliances for defects of the oral cavity.

Protrusional lisp: an articulation distortion usually of sibilant phonemes produced by the tongue being placed between the upper and lower teeth, suggestive of /th/ sounds.

Pseudohypacusis: apparent hearing impairment without an organic basis.

Psychoneurotic theory: a notion of the cause of stuttering, suggesting that the stutterer has an unconscious need or drive that the conscious mind finds quite unacceptable to express.

Pure agraphia: difficulties in writing.

Pure alexia: a condition in which the person cannot read, but retains normal writing, speech, and spoken language.

Pure tone: an auditory signal of a single frequency.

Pure-tone audiometry: auditory test in which a listener's minimum sensitivity (threshold) to pure tones is compared with that of the "average normal ear" at various frequencies.

Pure-tone threshold: the lowest stimulus intensity level of a specific frequency that can be detected roughly half of the time it is presented.

Pure word deafness: a type of aphasia in which the person does not recognize or repeat speech.

Quality disorders: resonance problems in voice, often hyponasality or hypernasality.

Rarefaction wave: an expanding area of decreased pressure immediately following a compressed wave as sound propagates through a medium.

Receptive aphasia: a language disorder due to brain injury or degeneration which causes loss of the ability to understand the meaning of words and sentences that are heard and may interfere with the person's ability to monitor his/her own speech.

Receptive language: the understanding of spoken or written messages by an individual.

Reflex arc: an involuntary physiologic (e.g., muscular) reaction to a sensory stimulus provided to the central nervous system, to interconnecting neural elements, and to efferent nerves to activate tissue.

Reissner's membrane: the thin wall separating the scala vestibuli from the scala media in the cochlea.

Remediation: activities for improvement that consider the nature of communication error, possible etiologic conditions, the overall character of the individual, and his/her ability to be stimulated to make changes.

Resonance: sympathetic or forced vibration of the air (i.e., sound) in the cavities beyond the source of a sound.

Resonance chambers: cavities in the vocal tract that modify laryngeal tone; the vestibule of the larynx, the laryngopharynx, the oropharynx, and the nasopharynx are some of the structures in which resonance occurs.

Resonance phenomena: the physical acoustic changes made in the original vocal tones, e.g., vowel sounds.

Respiratory tract: air passages from the nares into the lungs, including the nasal cavities, pharynx, larynx, trachea, and bronchi; allows passage of inhaled air into and exhaled air from the lungs, and provides adequate expiratory pressures to vibrate the vocal folds and an airstream from which vowel and consonant sounds can be produced.

Rochester method: a technique used in educating hearing-impaired children that combines speech expression and receptive skills through the auditory and speech channels with the use of fingerspelling.

Round window: an opening in the temporal bone at the base of the scala tympani in the cochlea; situated just below the oval window.

Scala media: cochlear space between the scala vestibuli and scala tympani, containing endolymph and the organ of Corti.

Scala tympani: cochlear space connecting with the scala vestibuli at the apex and the round window at the base; contains perilymph.

Scala vestibuli: cochlear space connecting with the scala tympani at the apex and the vestibule at the base; contains perilymph.

Semantics: the study of word expression and meaining.

Semitone: a half-step or half-interval part of a full interval or whole tone in a musical scale.

Sensation level: intensity of a stimulus in decibels above a person's auditory threshold, usually for that stimulus.

Sensorineural hearing impairment: decrement in hearing abilities resulting from damage to the auditory or neural sensory mechanism.

Sensorineural system: combines the "sensory" aspect of hair-cell excitation with the "neural" transmission of energy into the central system for auditory perception.

Sensory-perceptual ability: the auditory and cognitive potential to receive stimuli and to recognize them.

Sibilants: fricative sounds whose production is accompanied by a hissing noise.

Simultaneous method: "total communication" approach to educating hearing-impaired persons, combining the aural method with the use of fingerspelling and manual signs.

Sociocusis/socioacusis: decreased hearing due to exposure to noise other than that occurring at the workplace.

Soft palate: *see* Velum.

Somesthetic: conscious awareness of body sensation, e.g., pain, heat, touch.

Sound: an audible, organized movement of molecules in a medium.

Sound pressure level (SPL): a quantity of sound expressed by comparing the intensity of a particular sound with a standard intensity level.

Speech: the faculty of expressing thought by spoken words or sound symbols that are understood by another.

Speech audiometry: tests of auditory function using speech stimuli.

Speech conservation techniques: methods by which hearing-impaired individuals develop increased awareness of kinesthetic cues as the articulators and larynx are properly positioned for speech. Tactile and visual feedback channels supplement whatever audition remains.

Speech discrimination test: auditory test in which the listener identifies monosyllabic words presented at comfortably loud levels.

Speech disorder: unacceptable variations from the common form of speech creating negative impressions on the listener, lowered intelligibility, and personal disturbance in the speaker.

Speech frequencies: those frequencies commonly used in pure-tone audiometry that are most represented in a typical speech acoustic spectrum (500, 1000, and 2000 Hz).

Speech intelligibility: ability to accurately recognize a monosyllabic speech stimulus.

Speech-language pathologist: a specialist in the evaluation and nonmedical management of persons having disorders of speech and language.

Speech pathology: the field and profession concerned with evaluation of speech and language function or malfunction and amelioration of medically irreversible speech and language disorders.

Speechreading: act of recognizing the speech of others by visual observation of facial and bodily movements of the speaker.

Speech reception threshold (SRT): minimum intensity at which bisyllabic words or phrases (e.g., baseball, hot dog) can be correctly identified about half of the time they are presented.

Spondees: bisyllabic words used in establishing a speech reception threshold, such as "cowboy" and "ink well"; equal stress is placed on the pronunciation of each syllable.

Stapedectomy: a surgical procedure for the treatment of otosclerosis. The stapes and its footplate are removed, and ossicular chain continuity is restored with a prosthesis.

Stapes: one of the three bones (ossicles) in the middle ear; attached to the incus and to the oval window.

Stop: a type of consonant that is the result of the vocal system being arrested, or stopped; stops include /p/, /t/, /k/, /b/, /d/, and /k/.

Stroke: a cerebral-vascular accident that often leaves the individual with residual paralysis and brain function disorders.

Structure: the syntax and grammar of language (form).

Struggle behavior: forcing or prolonging the speech act by the stuttering child.

Stuttering: the disruption of the forward flow of speech, characterized by pauses, prolongations, and repetitions.

Substitution: errors in articulation in which a speech-sound other than the appropriate phoneme is produced.

Synapse: an interposed fluid gap between nerve fibers through which nerve impulses are transmitted, usually in the centers or nuclei, the gray matter of the nervous system.

Syntax: rule-directed order by which elements of language (e.g., words) can occur (grammar) in a sentence.

Tectorial membrane: gelatinous membrane in the scala media; part of the organ of Corti.

Telephone Devices for the Deaf (TDDs):   machines on which messages can be typed, sent simultaneously by telephone, and received as a visual display in standard English.

Temporal bone: the skull bone housing the auditory and vestibular systems.

Temporal lobe: midportion of the brain's cerebral cortex, serving audition; it generally serves audition.

Test reliability: a statement of surety concerning a test or instrument, indicating the degree of confidence in the test's repeatability.

Test validity: a statement of surety concerning the ability of a test to access or measure what it should.

Therapy: management of a significantly adverse condition to prevent, alleviate, or remove it.

Threshold: *see* Pure-tone threshold.

Tinnitus: auditory buzzing, hissing, or ringing sensations that are especially noticeable in quiet settings; most commonly associated with sensorineural conditions.

Tone: a sound characterized by a definite pitch or harmonic combination of pitches.

Tongue-thrust: the forward positioning of the tongue in speech, swallowing, or rest activities.

Tongue-tie: *see* Ankyloglossia.

Tonsils: masses of lymphoid tissue in the upper vocal tract, including the pharyngeal tonsil ("adenoid") in the nasal pharynx, palatine tonsil ("tonsil") between the oral cavity proper and the oral pharynx, and lingual tonsil over the posterior tongue surface.

Total communication method: *see* Simultaneous method.

Trachea: cartilaginous and membranous tubular part of the respiratory passageway that extends from the larynx through the thorax and divides into the bronchi, which enter the lungs.

Transcortical aphasia: disturbance of the initiation of speech or language stemming from damage of connections between brain centers serving speech and language functions.

Trauma: an injury to living tissue or functions.

Tympanic membrane (eardrum): a tough, three-layered structure situated at the end of the ear canal; forms the boundary between the outer and middle ear, and is considered a structure of the middle ear, serving to transfer airborne sound to middle-ear ossicles.

Tympanoplasty: plastic surgery repair of residual damage to the tympanic membrane and/or middle ear contents.

Unbound morpheme: smallest language unit carrying meaning.

Unilateral: associated with a single side.

Use: *see* Pragmatics.

Utterance: unit of spoken expression preceded and followed by silence; may be made up of words, phrases, clauses, or sentences.

Uvula: a highly variable structure that terminates the soft palate posteriorly.

Vagus nerve: cranial nerve X, parts of which serve sensory and motor functions to the pharynx and larynx.

Vascular disorders: abnormalities of the cardiovascular (blood circulatory) system; may be an occluded blood vessel or a sudden break in a vessel wall.

Velopharyngeal closure: separation of the nasopharynx from the oropharynx in speech and in swallowing by action of the muscles of the pharyngeal walls and the soft palate.

Velopharyngeal port: the opening between the oropharynx and nasopharynx.

Velum (soft palate): the posterior palate; largely muscular tissue separating the oral cavity from the nasal cavity.

Ventricular (false) folds: laryngeal structures above the vocal folds, usually functioning to protect the airway, but not involved in normal speech production; vestibular folds.

Verbal: pertaining to words, both spoken and written.

Vertigo: dizziness; a sensation of whirling or irregular motion, often associated with stimulation of the vestibular system.

Vestibular nerve: the branch of cranial nerve VIII related to the vestibular system and the sense of balance.

Vestibular system: system informing the brain of head position by the movement of fluid within the three semicircular canals embedded in the temporal bone and the stimulation of associated sensory cells.

Visemes: visual phonemes readily observed by the average listener in continuous speech.

Visual reinforcement audiometry: tests of a child's response to sounds that use conditioning of the child to look for the movement of an object (e.g., stuffed animal) after hearing a sound stimulus.

Vocal folds: paired structures in the larynx that act as valves against the entrance of foreign objects into the lower airway and lungs; during speech they vibrate against a forced stream of air, producing phonation; sometimes called vocal cords.

Vocalization: the production of voice.

Vocal nodules: small growths or neoplasms on one or both vocal folds interfering with the closure of the glottis and affecting the regularity of vocal fold vibrations; usually arising from vocal abuse.

Vocal tract: anatomic chambers from the larynx (vocal folds) to the pharynx and nasal and oral cavities; serving speech functions of phonation, resonance, articulation, and prosody.

Voice: in speech, sound produced by the vibration of the vocal folds and modified by the resonators.

Voice disorder: a disorder characterized by inappropriate pitch (too high, too low, never changed, or interrupted by breaks); loudness (too loud or not loud enough); or quality (harsh, hoarse, breathy, or nasal) (American Speech-Language-Hearing Association).

Voicing: one of the features in articulation describing the presence of phonation in phoneme production, as in voiced/voiceless consonants.

Vowels: phonemes produced by modifications of the vocal tone in a relatively unconstricted vocal tract, especially the oral cavity.

Wernicke's aphasia (syntactic aphasia): disorder in language use, although fluent and well-articulated; not making grammatical sense.

Wernicke's area: the language area of the left cerebral cortex toward the back of the brain in the superior temporal gyrus.

Index

Page numbers followed by "t" denote tables; those followed by "f" denote figures.